The First Survivors
of Alzheimer's

OTHER BOOKS BY DALE E. BREDESEN, MD

The End of Alzheimer's
The End of Alzheimer's Program

The

First Survivors

of

Alzheimer's

How Patients Recovered Life
and Hope in Their Own Words

DALE E. BREDESEN, MD

AVERY
an imprint of Penguin Random House
New York

AVERY

An imprint of Penguin Random House LLC
penguinrandomhouse.com

Most Avery books are available at special quantity discounts for bulk purchase for sales promotions, premiums, fund-raising, and educational needs. Special books or book excerpts also can be created to fit specific needs. For details, write SpecialMarkets@penguinrandomhouse.com.

Library of Congress Cataloging-in-Publication Data

Names: Bredesen, Dale E., author.
Title: The first survivors of Alzheimer's: how patients recovered life and hope in their own words / Dale Bredesen, MD.
Description: New York: Avery, Penguin Random House LLC, [2021] | Includes index.
Identifiers: LCCN 2021010967 (print) | LCCN 2021010968 (ebook) | ISBN 9780593192429 (paperback) | ISBN 9780593192436 (ebook)
Subjects: LCSH: Alzheimer's disease—Patients—Personal narratives.
Classification: LCC RC523.2 .B736 2021 (print) | LCC RC523.2 (ebook) | DDC 616.8/311—dc23
LC record available at https://lccn.loc.gov/2021010967
LC ebook record available at https://lccn.loc.gov/2021010968

Printed in the United States of America
3rd Printing

Book design by Laura K. Corless

This book is dedicated to Deborah, Kristin, Julie, Marcy, Sally, Edward, and Frank: your courage, diligence, and open-mindedness have paved the way for millions more survivors like you. Thank you on behalf of all of us.

CONTENTS

CONTENTS

Lost in Translation

If you want to go fast, go alone;
if you want to go far, go together.
—AFRICAN PROVERB

magine being told that you have Alzheimer's disease. Because this is such a common disease, there is a very good chance that this will happen to someone you love or someone I love. Now imagine that, instead of being told there is no hope, you are told that this is readily treatable, and that you can expect to get your normal cognition back; what's more, your children may be assured that they, their children, and your family's subsequent generations can avoid Alzheimer's disease. This reversal of fortune is life-changing, with reverberations through the generations ad infinitum. This was the goal in translating the research that my colleagues and I performed over thirty years into a therapeutic approach.

Do you remember the first time you heard that an untreatable illness had finally become treatable? Down through history, we humans have conquered one disease after another, often through biochemical research, sometimes through anecdotes from tribal medicine, and other times through sheer dumb luck. Regardless of the method, though, the result with each vanquished disease initially feels miraculous: suddenly the death sentences are lifted from thousands or even millions of people, restoring hope and a future for each. These events represent one of the most rewarding aspects of what it means to be human, and they never cease to inspire me:

Najiv was a teenage boy in the 1940s, living in a village in India, when he developed fever and a headache and lapsed into unconsciousness. He was taken by bullock cart from his village to the city, where the doctor diagnosed bacterial meningitis. At the time, this was typically a rapidly fatal illness. On this occasion, however, the doctor told Najiv's parents, "Until last week there would have been nothing I could do to save your son, but a new drug has just arrived from England. It is called penicillin." Instead of dying, then, Najiv made a full recovery, and this is of more than passing interest to all of us: Najiv's son is one of the most gifted biomedical researchers I have ever met, and his research may offer the best hope for an effective antiviral treatment not just for the COVID-19 of the current pandemic but also for any subsequent coronavirus pandemics—a brilliant advance with global lifesaving ramifications.

Whether it is Edward Jenner's development of the first vaccine—it has been pointed out that Jenner is responsible for saving more lives than any other human in history—or Frederick Banting and Charles Best's discovery of insulin, thus saving millions with diabetes, or David Ho's development of triple therapy to treat HIV effectively, each of these pioneers conjured hope from hopelessness, each sent a ripple through the reality we live with day to day, creating endless possibilities that did not hitherto exist, and altering the world's future irrevocably.

The seven survivors you'll read about here—in their own words—are pioneers as well. You'll hear from Kristin—the very first person who adopted our protocol ("Patient Zero")—who had watched her mother sink into dementia, and then was told by her own physician that she was on her way to suffering the same fate, without hope for treatment. How would each of us feel to receive such news from our physician? You'll also hear from Deborah, who suffered as her beloved father and grandmother were both lost to Alzheimer's, and then was horrified as she developed the same symptoms they had manifested, wondering what lay in store for her children. And from Edward, who was told to close his businesses and get his affairs in order. And Marcy, who piled up dozens of parking tickets because she could never remember to feed the parking meters. And Sally, a nurse educator who taught her students that medicine had no effective treatment to offer Alzheimer's patients, then developed it herself and failed a drug trial. And Frank, who had plans to write a book chronicling his own descent into dementia. And finally from Julie, who asked an expert neurologist if he could simply help her to avoid further decline and was told, "Good luck with that." The thoughts, concerns, emotions, and ultimate triumphs these survivors experienced are described with a depth of feeling that only those who lived them could express.

All of these pioneers are still on the trail—they survived "terminal" PET scans, MRI scans, family histories, and the prognostications of their physicians, thanks to their own inquisitiveness and industry to find a new solution, their courage to address the underlying drivers of their cognitive decline, and their determination to stick with a novel protocol.

Thanks to these first survivors, the way is now clear for the millions more in need, for both prevention and reversal of cognitive decline. These pioneers are catalyzing a paradigm shift in the way we think about, evaluate, prevent, and treat Alzheimer's disease and the pre-Alzheimer's conditions, MCI (mild cognitive impairment) and SCI (subjective cognitive impairment).

But why did it take so long? Alzheimer's disease was first described way back in 1906, yet the first survivors did not begin treatment until 2012, over a century later. Why so long? The fundamental difference between the way people were treated from 1906 until 2012 (and, unfortunately, the way most are still treated, unsuccessfully, today) and the therapeutics used for all of the survivors, is an obvious one: with all previous approaches, patients were given a Procrustean prescription for a single drug, such as Aricept, that has nothing to do with what is actually causing the cognitive decline.

In contrast, each of the survivors was evaluated for the various factors that were causing the decline itself, then those contributors were targeted with the personalized, precision medicine protocol we dubbed ReCODE (for "reversal of cognitive decline"). Some had undiagnosed infections—Marcy, for example, as you'll see from her story, had an undiagnosed infection from a tick bite, a relatively common one called ehrlichiosis, and treating that, along with her multiple other contributors, was important for best outcome; Sally, on the other hand, had exposure to mycotoxins (toxins produced by some molds), and removing her exposure was critical to her success. Each of the survivors you'll hear from had a different set of contributors, so that the optimal protocol for each survivor was different.

The notion that a complex chronic illness such as Alzheimer's disease should not be treated blindly, but instead should be treated by addressing the underlying drivers, may seem obvious. Attempting to treat Alzheimer's blindly is like trying to land a space capsule on the moon by pointing it in a random direction and crossing your fingers, yet that is exactly the standard of care at many Alzheimer's centers throughout the world. Why?

The answer lies in the African proverb "If you want to go fast, go alone; if you want to go far, go together." That is wonderful advice in many cases, but what happens when you do go together and you do indeed go very far—but it is in the *wrong direction*? Now, being together has borne you much farther from your goal than you were when you started, and is taking you farther and farther off course. But what amplifies this problem is that the group you are with keeps trying to convince itself that it *is* going in the right direction, despite all evidence to the contrary. Furthermore, the members of the group have all tied their livelihoods to this misdirection—with major fundraising, drug development, pharmaceutical fortunes, career-making publications, biotech start-ups, grant-approval power, self-congratulatory ceremonies, and on and on. Now it is virtually impossible to change course. What began idealistically as science and medicine has morphed into politics—and in politics, one of the least potent weapons is truth.

There is one piece of good news here—very good news, actually—which is that the basic research itself, the foundational research on which the development of Alzheimer's treatments rests, is quite solid, reproducible, and even elegant. A great deal has been learned about the pathology, epidemiology, microbiology, and biochemistry of Alzheimer's disease, and this has been published in well over 100,000 biomedical papers. So the tools we need to play chess with the Alzheimer's devil are available—the research is solid, the data are accurate, and we know a lot about the devil's strategy and moves. But the *translation* of all of these data into an effective treatment and prevention protocol is what has failed—miserably.

Because we have all followed this ultimately Gadarene march, the entire field of Alzheimer's treatment and prevention recommendations is completely backward! We are told by the experts not to check our genetic status for ApoE4, the most common genetic risk for Alzheimer's, because "there is nothing" we can do about it. But ask the more than 3,000 people on the website ApoE4.Info, who share their prevention strategies (the vast majority of whom are on some variation of the ReCODE Protocol we developed). We are told by the experts that "there is nothing that will prevent, reverse, or delay Alzheimer's disease." However, peer-reviewed publications from multiple groups contradict this claim.

We are told that mild cognitive complaints are "probably not Alzheimer's, so don't worry . . . and if it *is* Alzheimer's, there is nothing you can do anyway, so there is no need to come in early." This is the opposite of what we should do—in fact, the underlying changes in our brains begin about twenty years before a diagnosis of Alzheimer's, and there is a tremendous amount that can be done, for both prevention and reversal, just as these survivors discovered. The earlier you start, the easier it is to achieve improvement. And if you have cognitive complaints that do not turn out to be Alzheimer-related, you still want to have them treated successfully, of course!

So many of us are told that our memory complaints are "just part of normal aging," which allows Alzheimer's to sneak up on us and delays the very treatment we need. Often the physician says, "Come back next year, you're fine," annually, until finally one year, "Oh, it's Alzheimer's, we have no treatment except a drug that doesn't work." I cannot emphasize this strongly enough: when you are on an appropriate prevention or treatment, your aging should not be accompanied by cognitive problems—so-called age-related memory loss means that something is wrong. We can now identify the contributors and deal with them effectively—the earlier the better—and make dementia the rare condition it should be.

This idea that memory loss is just a part of normal aging is so pervasive that it delays our evaluations and leads to widespread misunderstanding. One of the patients who came to see me with "senior moments" was a superb physician who turned out to have Alzheimer's, as documented by amyloid PET scan, by FDG (fluorodeoxyglucose, which measures the brain's use of glucose) PET scan, and by MRI (magnetic resonance imaging). He also had a strong family history and genetic susceptibility with ApoE4. Despite all of that documentation, he was told that he was just displaying mild, age-related memory changes! However, his testing showed that he was bound for the nursing home if we did not intervene effectively. And he is now doing well, thankfully.

At the same time that the experts are telling us not to check our genetics, that there is nothing to be done, and that memory loss is just part of normal aging, most are *failing* to tell us what is arguably the most important point: the children of those who suffer from memory loss should be evaluated as they reach their 40s and should begin a targeted prevention protocol, so that they can end the memory loss with the current generation. But when was the last time your doctor explained this to you and offered to do the appropriate evaluation for each child?

Everything about the evaluation, prevention, and treatment of cognitive decline is completely backward, and it's not just what our doctors are telling us but also how we respond—I can't tell you how many times I've heard from a patient that "It's not that bad—my spouse isn't so great, either." There is an old joke about such an elderly couple. Husband Bob says to wife Sadie, "I'm concerned about your memory, so I'm going to give you a little memory test: can you go to the kitchen and make two eggs over easy, hash browns, three strips of bacon, and one cup of black coffee?" Sadie laughs. "Heck, that's easy," she says, and trots off to the kitchen. Bob hears pots and pans banging, then about fifteen minutes later, out comes Sadie, proudly carrying a parfait glass filled with ice cream topped with fudge and whipped cream and sprinkled with nuts. Bob cocks his head, shoots her a quizzical look, and gripes, "Hey, you forgot the cherry!" So if both your spouse and you are exhibiting memory loss, it doesn't mean you don't need evaluation— it means you *both* need evaluation! And as you might imagine, couples who both follow the protocol often help each other with compliance, making things easier for each other.

The experts also tell us that "promising drugs are in the pipeline." We have been hearing this for decades. In 1980 we were told there should be something effective by 1990; in 1990 we were told there should be something by 2000; and on and on it goes. Over 400 clinical trials have now failed. Because the party line is that the amyloid that collects in the brains of patients with Alzheimer's causes the disease, billions of dollars have been spent developing and testing antibodies ("mabs," short for "monoclonal antibodies") that remove the amyloid. One after the other after the other, these have all failed to improve cognition in patients with Alzheimer's: from bapineuzumab to solanezumab to crenezumab to gantenerumab, and most recently, aducanumab.

Aducanumab was considered to be the most promising Alzheimer's drug candidate in years, and it led to an increase in the value of the stock of its pharmaceutical company, Biogen, by billions of dollars. This is not surprising, because a truly successful Alzheimer's drug—something for which there is inarguably a dire need—is likely to be a $100 billion drug. But at what point do the financial stakes become so incredibly high that the rational thinking and analysis required for best patient outcomes is clouded? At what point does the cash register become so heavy that it crushes the patient? Perhaps you may judge for yourself: after two clinical trials failed, the FDA rejected approval for aducanumab. Normally this would end the application process, as it has for so many other drug candidates. But the potential for $100 billion is very difficult to walk away from, so an internal statistician—one employed by Biogen—"reanalyzed" the data. Lo and behold, the Biogen statistician found what the external, impartial statistician had not—that aducanumab should be approved after all. (Shortly after the "reanalysis," the statistician left the company. He claimed that this had nothing to do with the reanalysis.)

And why did he believe it should be approved? Not because it improved patients' cognition—no one is suggesting that aducanumab improves cognition in patients with Alzheimer's disease. Not because it stopped the cognitive decline—it did not. Instead, the argument is that it may have slowed the decline in cognition slightly. In one study, it showed no such effect, whereas in another study, at one dose but not another, it did show a slowing of decline. So it either had no effect or almost no effect. However, that was enough for Biogen to bully—er, I mean, request—that the FDA reconsider approval.

The FDA acceded to Biogen's request for reconsideration, but before its team of external reviewers met, the FDA released a "smoke signal" statement suggesting that the drug would be approved, stating that "there is substantial evidence of effectiveness to support approval." As you might well imagine, Biogen's stock soared, adding nearly $20 billion to the company's value! However, just two days later—barely enough time for the champagne to lose its fizz—a panel of experts not affiliated with Biogen criticized the FDA sharply for releasing the smoke signal that implied an upcoming approval and voted overwhelmingly to recommend to the FDA that it deny approval of the drug. This led to a Biogen stock plunge of 31 percent, reducing the company's value by $19 billion. After causing such a huge financial loss—which has happened before, following previous results for the same drug—aducanumab is threatening to become the Bernie Madoff of Alzheimer's drugs.

If you think it smells fishy that the FDA released a statement hinting at approval before the expert panel of analysts met, then hold your nose, because it gets worse. In an unusual move, the FDA, which usually sends out two different reviews of each drug candidate—one by the FDA itself (intended to be impartial, of course) and another by the company (which is understandably biased toward approval)—mixed the two reports in a single report! This move left even the used-car salesmen laughing and shaking their heads.

But here's the punch line: despite the strong negative recommendation from the experts, the failed trial, and the previous rejection, the FDA could *still* approve aducanumab (yes, you read that correctly), ignoring the vehement criticisms of the panel of experts. In fact, some foundations have suggested approval despite the lack of proven efficacy—which is like saying, "Okay, I know that this parachute does not work, but I'd like to wear it on the way down anyway. And I'll pay a hundred billion dollars for it."

Ironically, these antibodies designed to reduce amyloid may turn out to be quite valuable in the treatment of Alzheimer's when used in a completely different way. Instead of trying to remove the amyloid without removing the various insults that are causing your brain to produce the amyloid—the chronic infections, the prediabetes, the vascular damage, the toxins, etc.—if the antibodies were used to remove the amyloid *after* these various insults had been withdrawn and the metabolism optimized, then it would actually make sense.

So as you can see, the translation of Alzheimer's research into effective treatment and prevention has failed, and because of that, the recommendations for those at risk or exhibiting symptoms make little sense. The future involves a fundamentally different approach, directed at determining all of the factors contributing to cognitive decline and then targeting those with a personalized, precision medicine approach. It is the approach that resulted in the first survivors, who now number in the many hundreds. I did not suggest this new approach, nor reject the classical teaching on Alzheimer's lightly, but after thirty years of research, I realized something did not make sense.

A LESSON FROM DISNEYLAND

As a freshman in college, I had become fascinated by the brain, and after studying its anatomy, physiology, and chemistry, I wanted to understand how diseases like Alzheimer's, Parkinson's, and Huntington's affect the normal workings of the brain. When the brain is impacted by various diseases, surprising symptoms appear that reveal the inner workings of our neural systems: some people completely lose the ability to fall asleep, in a disease called fatal familial insomnia; others fling their limbs while dreaming, often injuring their spouses, in a condition called REM sleep behavior disorder; still others become convinced that their spouse has been replaced by an impostor, in a condition known as Capgras syndrome.

However, medical school really brought home the sad reality of what it is to work with patients with brain disease. The term *healer* had to be taken quite loosely in neurology, since it was mostly about diagnostics, not therapeutics. Medical school rotations on obstetrics brought us happy mothers and miracle babies; thoracic surgery brought us healed hearts; and even oncology brought us cancer survivors. But I could see why my classmates did not want to become neurologists. Ninety-nine percent of being a brain doctor was not about making people better, but about diagnosing what it was that you could *not* help them with, from Alzheimer's to Lou Gehrig's to frontotemporal dementia and on and on. We watched helplessly as the intricate neural networks that confer humanness on each patient decomposed before our eyes. It became clear that the area of greatest medical treatment failure was in these neurodegenerative diseases. I hoped that learning more about them as a neurology resident and then as a neuroscientist would shed some light on why.

Paradoxically, the experts in neurology taught me expertise in failure—learning to color inside the lines when nothing inside the lines had ever worked was perhaps not the best strategy. The experts simply parroted the phrase "There is nothing that can prevent, reverse, or delay Alzheimer's disease." This was considered a fundamental principle, not to be challenged. As the Greek philosopher Epictetus said, "It is impossible to begin to learn that which one thinks one already knows." Thus we focused on diagnostics, on neuroanatomy and neurophysiology, on neurochemistry and neurogenetics—everything except novel approaches to therapeutics. Over the years, I gave up on the idea of healing and focused on being a neurologist.

After all of my many years of training, I had been so inculcated with the knowledge that neurodegenerative diseases are terminal illnesses, impossible to treat, that I had become an expert in failure. As Walt Disney observed, there are two types of people: the "yes if" people and the "no because" people. The "no because" people can always give you a long list of reasons that any new idea is doomed to failure; whereas the "yes if" people will point out that, if you'll take specific considerations into account, your idea just might have a chance at success. Thus was Disneyland born, but so, too, the moon landing, the internet, and virtually every other notable advance.

I realized that I had become a "no because" person, an expert armed with a myriad of finely honed, abstrusely technical, academically sophisticated details explaining why nothing could be done for those suffering with Alzheimer's. I had become an ordained minister of the Church of No Hope. I explained to each suffering family member that the Alzheimer's Emperor was draped in the Clothes of Impossibility, and even though they might not be able to see them, as an expert I could assure them that they were indeed there. To say this work was dispiriting would be an understatement.

Therefore, I decided to give up the hopelessness of the neuro-degeneration clinics—indeed, I did not see a patient for twenty years—and set up a laboratory to study the fundamental biochemical mechanisms that drive the death of brain cells and their synaptic connections. What goes wrong? How does it start? Why is it so common? The idea was to return to the clinic if my lab group and I could ever find anything of promise.

So the good news and bad news here are the same: because of the well over 100,000 papers published on Alzheimer's disease, virtually any new theory can be rejected quickly, based on what has already been published. Indeed, it is nearly impossible to come up with a theory that satisfies all of the many findings already published. Maybe Alzheimer's really is an impossible disease to treat successfully?

I considered the future: At some point, perhaps fifty or a hundred years down the road, some group would come up with an accurate model of Alzheimer's disease that would explain the many disparate findings from epidemiological studies to genetic studies to pathological studies, and, critically, would predict an effective treatment and explain the many failed treatments. What would that group think of that we hadn't? What mold would that group break that we hadn't?

All of the previous theories explained little pieces of the overall picture—some explained pieces of the genetics, some parts of the pathology, some parts of the epidemiology, for example—but none was compatible with all of the findings. Most important, none had ever led to an effective treatment.

We considered what a successful theory would need to explain:

- Why do the many risk factors seem to have no connection—from reduced vitamin D to reduced estrogen to chronic infections to high homocysteine to cardiovascular disease to sleep apnea to systemic inflammation to mercury exposure and on and on?

- Why do some people collect large amounts of the Alzheimer's-associated amyloid, yet have no cognitive decline, whereas others suffer cognitive decline with little or no amyloid?

- How does ApoE4—a genetic risk carried by 75 million Americans—create such risk for Alzheimer's?

- Why does Alzheimer's risk increase dramatically with aging?

- Why does Alzheimer's start where it does in the brain— often in a specific area of the temporal lobe—and spread as it does?

- Why is Alzheimer's associated with plastic regions of the brain—regions that are associated with learning and memory?

- Why has drug treatment for Alzheimer's failed?

- Of highest priority, how can we tackle Alzheimer's treatment successfully?

Fast-forward a few decades of observing brain cells dying in a petri dish, using fruit flies to create "Alzflymer's" and transgenic mice to create "Mouzheimer's," and testing many thousands of compounds to identify an optimal drug candidate . . . all of the thousands and thousands of experiments led us to some shocking conclusions:

- **The heart and soul of Alzheimer's disease—its most fundamental nature—is a chronic or repeated** *insufficiency.* Not a simple insufficiency like vitamin C deficiency, which leads to scurvy, but rather an insufficiency in a neuroplasticity network, a brain network that changes with learning and memory—not misfolded proteins, not amyloid, not tau, not prions, not reactive oxygen species—these are all mediators of the response to the insufficiency, not the cause—but an insufficiency in a neuroplasticity network. This is something like having an entire nation enter a recession—there are many potential contributors, and these must be identified and rectified to end the recession. To extend the analogy, the coronavirus is a *cause* of the recession (the major contributor), whereas staying home is a *mediator*: in order to end the recession, we need to eradicate the coronavirus (or become immune to it)—simply leaving home will leave the cause unchecked, and thus fail to solve the problem.

- This neuroplasticity network requires many factors to function optimally, from hormones to nutrients to growth factors to oxygenated blood flow to energy—but also requires an absence of infections, toxins, and inflammation for efficient operation.

* The amyloid and tau that have been vilified in Alzheimer's disease are actually part of the *protective response* to the insults that create the insufficiency, and therefore, targeting them with drugs is of little help unless you first identify and remove the various insults and quell the insufficiency.

These conclusions suggested a completely different treatment strategy from anything that had been tried before. Instead of treating with a single drug that would be the same for each person, we needed to flip the script: evaluate each person for all of the different parameters required for the network to function—the hormones, nutrients, infections, etc.—and then target the ones found to be suboptimal. Therefore, in 2011, we proposed the first comprehensive trial for Alzheimer's disease. Unfortunately, we were turned down by the IRB (institutional review board, which determines whether human clinical trials are allowed to be carried out) because we were proposing a new type of clinical trial that would test an algorithm, a personalized approach that depended on what was causing the cognitive decline, rather than testing a single drug. Getting turned down by the IRB was very depressing. How would we ever be able to determine whether this approach was on the right track?

Shortly after that, I received a call from the person who would become Patient Zero—which was somewhat surprising since I had not seen a patient in twenty years. However, although Patient

Zero—Kristin—lived a few thousand miles away, she had a friend from the San Francisco Bay Area who had gotten wind of our research. Kristin changed the world of Alzheimer's, and you can read about how she did this—and how six others did, as well—in their own words, on the following pages.

PART ONE

It Tolls for Thee No More:
The First Survivors
Tell Their Own Stories

CHAPTER 1

Kristin's Story:
Zero Is Far from Nothing

Necessity is the mother of invention.

—PLATO

Desperation is the dominatrix of disruption.

—NOT PLATO

Journal entry 2011

I know that I am on that slippery slope into Alzheimer's and I am terrified. My short-term memory is gone. Thoughts fly out of my head seconds after they form. I can't deny or hide it any longer. I feel lost. My heart is in my throat. I can't swallow. My ears are ringing. I'm hyperventilating. Seeing these words in my journal makes it real. My brain is slipping away. I'm really scared. The train is out of the station and it's going downhill without brakes.

I unlock the file drawer and take out the bag of sleeping pills I've collected over the past two years. I've kept each prescription in its original container to keep track of the expiration dates. I want them to work when the time comes. But it's not time, not yet. I have things to do before I die. I only hope that I will have courage to act and that I will do so before I no longer know how or when to do it.

I put the pills away and lock the drawer.

That scary passage from my diary reminds me of how far I've come. Reading it is painful, but doing so keeps me focused on the importance of staying on my path. This glimpse into my story is a testament to the success of ReCODE, the Bredesen Protocol. Without the protocol I would not be able to express my thoughts or write about them, and, I am sure, I would not even be alive today. I have mixed feelings about telling my story. I've procrastinated miserably writing this because remembering the details, especially reliving my feelings, brings back the fear. Even with my amazing success in reversing cognitive impairment, the terror of what almost was grabs me by the throat and squeezes the breath out of me. But here I go with the hope that sharing my story will help others and perhaps dispel some of the skepticism.

In the weeks that passed after that journal entry, I grew progressively worse. Deeply depressed and feeling at the end of my rope, I called my best friend and told her what I was planning. She knew about the years I'd spent caring for my mother during her long battle with Alzheimer's. She had heard me swear that I would not put my family through that pain if I was to get the disease. My friend was upset to hear me talking about ending my life. She told me about a research doctor she knew in California who was working on a cure for Alzheimer's. She reached out to Dr. Bredesen, set up an appointment, and insisted that I fly to California to meet with him. Despite my skepticism, I agreed. I was desperate to find a way to save my brain.

The Buck Institute for Research on Aging sits high on a hill overlooking the rolling landscape of beautiful Marin County, north of San Francisco. I was nervous. I had no idea of the challenging journey that lay ahead, but I was eager to try anything that would stop the progression of the disease. The receptionist directed me to Dr. Bredesen's office. I carried a small notebook because I knew I would forget anything that I didn't write down. I listened intently to Dr. Bredesen as he enthusiastically described his research—work he had dedicated his life to for over thirty years. He asked me about my situation and why I'd come to see him. Time flew by. We talked for hours while he described his theory and the background leading up to his recent discoveries. I understand it now, but at that time my brain was too damaged to process the information. But Dr. Bredesen's simple analogy of the damaged brain being comparable to a leaky roof with thirty-six holes that needed to be plugged one by one made sense. He explained that Alzheimer's is not one disease manifestation that a drug can fix but is rather a combination of numerous factors that have gone wrong. Most of the issues he described applied to me, some of which I was not aware of at that time. I told Dr. Bredesen that I was committed to following whatever he recommended. I knew he was my only hope. I left his office with a fire in my belly, determined to let nothing stand in my way of following the protocol. I was more than ready to get started.

At that time, I did not fully comprehend that I was the first patient to test his protocol. I have come to appreciate being known as Patient Zero. As other patients went on the protocol, our group grew to ten. Nine of us were able to reverse cognitive impairment. A truly remarkable success given that until then no treatment had reversed cognitive decline in Alzheimer's disease. Dr. Bredesen published the results of that small sample of ten in 2014. Since then, hundreds of successful reversals have been documented using the Bredesen Protocol. I am honored to have been the first!

By the end of our meeting, I had the basics of the protocol scribbled in my notebook, and for the first time, I felt optimistic that maybe I had a future that included a working brain. Dr. Bredesen advised me to follow the protocol under the supervision of a physician. That proved to be a challenge. Physicians were skeptical, especially neurologists. For the most part, their approach to treating people with impaired memory was to prescribe pharmaceutical drugs, knowing that those drugs offer nothing more than short-term improvements for some, and harsh side effects for many. In my mother's case, Aricept seemed to make her worse, and the side effects were harsh. I had no intention of taking the drugs. What's worse, doctors are often dismissive and sometimes rude when patients refuse the drugs and ask about alternative approaches. Luckily, I found a family doctor who was willing to give the protocol a chance. She also agreed to order the many lab tests Dr. Bredesen needed to monitor my progress. I kept in frequent contact with Dr. Bredesen. We tweaked the protocol when certain supplements caused undesired reactions. I had retinal scans to determine the level of amyloid plaque buildup I had in my brain. I gave feedback to Dr. Bredesen when certain activities made me feel especially focused, like exercise and yoga.

Here is another of my journal entries from the "dark days" before starting on the protocol:

I can no longer remember numbers—not my phone number, street number, family birthdays; often I forget what year it is. I seem to be stuck in the late 1900s. Yesterday I dated a check

1978. Bills go unpaid even when I have money in my account. My credit score is getting trashed. Utility companies are threatening to shut off service. I make foolish decisions, spending money unwisely for things I don't need. I get lost when I drive at night. I am forgetting the names of my pets. I am reaching for the light switch on the wrong wall! I forgot how to spell my grandchildren's names. Before they come to visit, I stare at their photos on my refrigerator and repeat their names and ages so I will remember when they arrive. Even that does not help. My youngest grandson runs to me with his little arms spread wide. I scoop him up for a hug, and to my horror, call him by his older brother's name. I struggle to find words. I substitute easier words. I can't spell, even four-letter words! I can't speak properly. I use the wrong words, using the incorrect but a similar-sounding word. I keep a small dictionary in my purse. I must look up simple familiar words. I get lost driving to familiar places and spend hours trying to find my parked car. All this scares the hell out of me.

DOWN THE RABBIT HOLE

Two startling events jolted me to the reality that I was no longer able to maintain my business. I was on a transcontinental flight. In my usual state of exhaustion, I fell asleep briefly, and when I woke up, I could not remember why I was flying to Dallas or whom I was supposed to meet. The more I racked my brain trying to remember, the more frustrated I became. Frantically I searched my briefcase for clues and found none. When the plane landed, I

7

booked the next flight home. A few weeks after that incident I was in a client's office presenting findings from a recent overseas assessment. As I stood in front of the group, in the middle of the presentation my mind went completely blank. I froze and could not remember what to say next. The polite group tapped their pens on the table for what seemed like an eternity. One woman tried to spark my memory by recapping the discussion. I was mortified. I could hear the blood rushing through my head in loud gurgles. I could not breathe. I rushed out of the room.

Within a short time, I lost my ability to understand technical reports, let alone write them. I had a reputation for researching and producing excellent work. Newspapers were next. I found myself reading and rereading the same sentences because I could not retain the meaning of what I had just read. I became deeply depressed. It was obvious that I could not represent myself as an expert in anything. I stopped working. I could no longer read a book!

Since childhood I had been an avid and rapid reader. I devoured books. Reading was my salvation growing up. I could escape to fantastic places far away from my crazy family and our poor existence. I mention this because it is an important part of who I became and the type of driven person I grew into. I was fiercely determined to improve my life, to rise above the poverty and abuse. I knew education was the avenue I would have to take. I worked two jobs after school to save money. As soon as I was out of high school, I bought a one-way ticket to New York and realized the dream I had nurtured from age 13.

Barely 17, I arrived with $60, four dresses sewn by my mother, and a burning passion to succeed in the Big Apple! I landed a job and enrolled in night classes at New York University. I spent weekends visiting New York's museums and concerts absorbing as much culture as I could, trying to make up for my lack of exposure to art and music growing up. I succeeded in all my endeavors and lived life at a whirlwind pace. I learned to fly and opened an aerial photography service in addition to my other businesses. I slept as few hours as I could get away with. I paid the price years later when my brain began to deteriorate.

I started experiencing brain fog in my late 40s when I was in perimenopause. My emotions were up and down. Despite a monetarily successful life, a marriage, a child, and a successful business, I could not dial down the pace or the resulting stress. The foggy thinking wasn't constant at that stage. It came and went, occurring most often when I was exhausted, sleep deprived, or highly stressed. I went back to school for a master's degree while working full time. Later I went on to earn a doctorate. More changes, including an amicable divorce, and with two more degrees in hand I began working overseas.

World traveler, independent, workaholic, multitasker—working in the world's most dangerous countries, trying to solve the problems of the world's poorest people, I was always in demand for the next assignment. I became an expert in my field. Living and working in harsh and stressful environments, I boasted that I didn't need to sleep—three to four hours a night was typical. I frequently stayed up all night to meet deadlines. I ate what was convenient, and it usually wasn't good for me. I battled serious parasitic infestations and tropical diseases with strong medicines, including antibiotics. I lived in moldy, water-damaged buildings while overseas in many locations. I didn't know at the time how harmful that was to my brain or, as I discovered later, that I am among the 24 percent of the population with a genetic makeup that cannot process the mold toxins. The negative effects were cumulative.

I realized how seriously mold affected me after an incident in Afghanistan. I was staying in an old house that had been unoccupied for years during the war. I pried open a kitchen cabinet in search of a teapot. The stuck door popped open. The pungent odor was so powerful that it literally knocked me backward and took away my breath. A solid layer of black mold lined the inside of the cabinet. I had a violent reaction to that extreme mold exposure. The sensitivity to mold gets worse with every exposure. I am sure that mold contributed significantly to my memory loss. Thanks to the excellent work of Dr. Ritchie Shoemaker (author of *Surviving Mold*), I have been able to detox from mold. Dr. Bredesen addressed the effects of exposure to toxic elements, including mold, with his typology of inhalational as one form of Alzheimer's. In my case, I have a combination of the types he identified.

I grew up in an athletic family and was a runner. Despite having healthy practices in my youth, I let go of most of them as an adult. I was obsessed with staying thin. I tried every new diet. I once ate only grapes for three days! I drank too much alcohol, took tranquilizers, and consumed copious quantities of coffee and diet soda to keep going. My emotions swung from exuberant, on the mountaintop, ready to conquer the world, down to the depths of despair, feeling like a worthless, incompetent fraud. My personal life reflected the wild surges and inconsistencies.

I blamed my memory problems on stress. I thought when I gave up my business and reduced the stress, I would get my brain back. But that didn't happen. I became aware that I was not joining in conversations as I had always done. I didn't have much to say. I couldn't think fast enough to join in a meaningful way, so I sat quietly. My thoughts were like fireflies caught in a jar, a brief illumination and then gone. Since I lived alone, I was able to keep my problem a secret, or so I thought. Later, after I began my recovery, I asked my son if he had noticed that anything was wrong with me. He said of course, but he didn't want to make me feel bad by mentioning it. He was very worried, having watched my mother slowly change from a dynamic businesswoman and loving grandmother into a person who could not recognize her family or even speak to them.

GETTING MY BRAIN BACK

With Dr. Bredesen's protocol in hand, and his assurance that he would be there for me, telling me I could reach out to him as I needed to, I returned home feeling optimistic. I was passionately committed to strict compliance, with no exceptions.

I visited my doctor, explained the protocol, and asked her to order the tests Dr. Bredesen recommended. I cleared out most of the food in my kitchen to make room for a new eating regimen. I bought supplements and started buying organic food. I had followed a vegetarian diet for several years, but it wasn't particularly healthy and included a lot of junk food. I started exercising more, at first three times a week at the gym. Then I rediscovered yoga, motivated at first as a means of decreasing stress and increasing sleep. I became a certified yoga instructor and a yoga therapist. A daily yoga practice is essential for me to maintain a healthy brain.

Changing lifelong poor sleep habits proved to be very difficult. Even as a child I didn't sleep enough. I went to bed late, woke up early, and often had nightmares that interrupted my sleep. It was to be one of my biggest challenges of the protocol—patching up the "insufficient sleep hole in my leaky roof." I usually had no trouble falling asleep but would wake up after just a few hours and stay awake for the rest of the night. I was more exhausted in the morning than when I went to bed. After going on the protocol, it took me over a year to begin to enjoy a full night's sleep of 7 to 7.5 hours. At this point, I am looking forward to the future when I may be able to sleep a full 8 hours or more! I learned that the brain cleanses itself of toxins during sleep and only during optimum sleep cycles. I had cheated my brain of that period of cleansing for most of my life.

I put a lot of effort into improving my sleep, and it has paid off. I keep the bedroom cool and dark. I removed all electronic equipment, electric clocks, internet modems, and television from my bedroom. I turn off my cell phone and do not place it near my head. I take time-released melatonin 30 minutes before bed. I do not use electronic devices an hour before bedtime. At night I read printed books instead of an e-book. I bought special glasses to neutralize the blue light if I am reading earlier in the evening. Once in bed, I use eye shades to shut out any ambient light. I put a sleep app on my phone called Insight Timer. It has a huge selection of guided meditations for sleep. The app helps me get back to sleep after I get up to go to the bathroom. Listening to the meditations keeps my mind from ruminating on daily problems, as I used to do. I've taught myself to navigate bathroom trips without turning on the light, sometimes keeping my eyes nearly closed. I made sure there are no obstacles to trip over between my bed and the bathroom. I look forward to going to sleep in the sacred space I created.

Changing eating habits was another major challenge. Fortunately, I love vegetables, olive oil, and butter, so switching to gluten-free, high-fat, low-carbohydrate, moderate-protein foods works well for me. Some years back when the food industry—and doctors—promoted the low-fat craze, I embraced it wholeheartedly. Nearly everything I bought was labeled low-fat. I read labels searching for fat content but paid no attention to the potential harm that sugar, artificial sweeteners, additives, and all the other junk in processed food inflicts. It was no wonder that I suffered from digestive issues—especially bloating after meals and indigestion. At one point, an internist put me on medication for GERD, those horrible purple pills that are so widely prescribed but have very harmful side effects, particularly for women prone to osteoporosis. I did not follow a gluten-free low-carb diet when I first went on the protocol. But I gave up sugar and artificial sweeteners. Once I tried the diet and stopped eating gluten, I could not believe how much better I felt. No more bloating and no cravings! And I lost seventeen pounds over about six months. My energy returned, but most important, the fog lifted from my brain and I could think again!

At the same time, I waged a war against inflammation and exposure to neurotoxins—especially mold in my case. I have detoxed my system and eliminated mold in my home, but I am concerned that mold spores still live in my body because of the violent reaction I have when in proximity to moldy environments.

Around age 40, I began to have arthritic pain in my hands and knees. Most mornings I woke up so stiff I had to walk downstairs sideways to keep from bending my knees too deeply. After being on the protocol a year, I realized the arthritis had disappeared! I believe the turmeric/curcumin supplement eliminated the inflammation in my joints as well as in my brain. That is a wonderful unexpected benefit for me. I now run up and down the stairs and have no pain in my hands or anywhere else in my body. I am more flexible than most people half my age.

In addition to taking the supplements recommended on the ReCODE Protocol, I shield myself from harmful substances to the extent possible. I drink only filtered water out of glass or stainless steel. I do not use plastic containers or aluminum. I eat whole foods, organic when possible, and do not buy processed foods. I eat gluten-free and lean toward a ketogenic diet with high fats, medium protein, and low carbohydrates. I fast 10 hours or more between dinner and breakfast. I periodically fast 24 hours, consuming only water. I use anti-inflammatory spices like cinnamon (a quarter teaspoon a day), cayenne pepper, black pepper, and turmeric. I maintain good dental hygiene by brushing and flossing often and getting frequent cleanings. I buy safe household products and clean with basic supplies like white vinegar and baking soda. I challenge my brain by taking graduate level courses in difficult subjects like neurology. I constantly research scientific articles on neuroscience and dementia. I teach at a major East Coast university, which keeps me on my toes—I have to read and lecture on all the papers I assign my students. I also teach an early morning yoga class and do a daily home yoga practice. In addition, I do aerobic exercise for 45 minutes a day four to five times a week, either on a treadmill or biking. I meditate 20 minutes twice a day and get at least 7 to 7.5 hours of sleep a night. I keep stress at a minimum. I socialize with friends and family often. And—critically—I maintain a positive attitude.

It is important to reiterate that the recovery process is a slow one. My foggy thinking and memory lapses did not disappear quickly. Recovery unfolded gradually. On several occasions, I was taken by surprise by how different I felt—the veil of murkiness was lifting. Thoughts started coming easily and in an orderly fashion. I began to read again and comprehend what I was reading. My brain was so sharp one morning that I ran through the house shouting, "I can think, my brain is back!" The clarity felt so different and unfamiliar. Clear thinking wasn't an experience that I felt constantly in the early days of my treatment—it came and went—but over time the periods of clarity lasted longer. I found I was easily handling tasks that I had been struggling with, like dealing with finances, bill paying, and planning. I wasn't having to go back to the first paragraph of an article over and over again. I noticed that I was listening to people when they spoke, really hearing what they were saying and being able to follow the conversation and respond appropriately. I began to read books again. I wasn't struggling to find the right word as often when speaking.

Fatigue and stress are enemies of clear thinking, and for me, reminders of my brain's fragility and the need to stay vigilant to protect it by staying on the protocol. I am terrified of slipping backward, so I've learned to guard against becoming too tired or stressed. Yoga and daily meditation have helped tremendously in that regard. Even though I became an advanced certified yoga teacher, I still need to take classes. As a teacher, I am focusing on the students. As a yoga student, I focus on my practice. It is the mind-body connection that comes with the poses and full breathing that brings relaxation and harmony to mind and body simultaneously. Oxygen and blood flow to the brain increase. I believe that new brain cells are formed during yoga as one goes through the poses and coordinated breathing. There are so many other benefits derived from yoga, including spiritual peace, balance, increased mobility, and lubrication of joints. Just do it!

I needed to get back to work. After about ten months into the protocol, I felt ready to accept a short-term consulting assignment. That was scary because it involved overseas travel to a stressful environment, and I knew it would disrupt my routine. It would mean greater challenges finding the right food and avoiding gluten. Minimizing sleep deprivation during and after 14- to 18-hour flights was not easy. I planned stopovers to allow an overnight stay to avoid loss of sleep. Sleep masks and earplugs are essential. I found that aerobic exercise upon arrival helps to reset the body clock.

Despite good planning, I had a setback. My first assignment was extended beyond the original commitment and I ran out of supplements. Work was stressful due to poor security, and I wasn't sleeping enough. I began to have periods of brain fog. The combination of lack of supplements, inadequate sleep, and stress resulted in a setback in my recovery. That was a major wake-up call. It clearly illustrated the importance of staying on the program. After I had been home for a couple of weeks, I was able to get back to where I had been before the trip.

A bout with the flu sent me backward briefly. I became too ill to eat, take supplements, exercise, or even meditate for nearly two weeks. I had to work my way back from that event as well. The major take-home lesson: The protocol is a process toward healing many aspects of dementia, but in order to hold on to the successes, it must be maintained with a total commitment to a new lifestyle!

I repeat, healing the brain after years of neglect and abuse doesn't happen overnight. The damage took place insidiously over many years before reaching the point of noticeable cognitive impairment. Even though I began to experience many positive improvements within a few months of going on the protocol, reversing memory loss is an ongoing process. The work never stops. I don't feel like I'm "cured," even though my Alzheimer's disease (AD) symptoms have reversed. I function at least as well as—and in many instances, far better than—I ever have in my life. Essentially the ReCODE Protocol boils down to adhering to major lifestyle changes. Keeping on the protocol day in and day out—continuous compliance—has been the hardest thing I have ever done. But I keep doing it because I am afraid not to. I'm afraid the disease will come back, and if it does, I might not be able to beat it back again. So I swallow the supplements, eat organic whole food, eliminate sugar and simple carbohydrates, meditate twice a day, do yoga and aerobics and lift weights, make sure I sleep well, stay calm, and socialize with humans and animals.

Given the complexities of the disease and the varying stages in which a person starts the protocol, the outcome can't be guaranteed. Does the protocol work for everyone? Sadly, it doesn't. The reasons may include the degree of cognitive decline when one starts the protocol or other mysteries of the disease yet to be unraveled. Some people, regardless of their fear of Alzheimer's, will not stay on the protocol. But to succeed, you must stick to it. Sometimes it is one step forward and two backward. As I said earlier, it takes time! Half measures get you nowhere with this protocol. I now coach people who follow the protocol under the care of a physician. With all the components of healing the brain, a coach is necessary because doctors don't have the time to guide the patient through the treatment. When my clients complain about giving up sugar, gluten, and starchy vegetables, I tell them to volunteer at an Alzheimer's care facility and then decide if they are willing to do all that is necessary to heal their brains. I think compliance is easier for those of us who have watched a parent slowly succumb to the disease. We know well what the future holds if we let down our guard.

The miracle turnaround that began when I met Dr. Bredesen

nine years ago continues on a day-to-day basis. A more willing patient would have been hard to find. I was so desperate I would have eaten dirt if I thought doing so would have given me back my brain! As it turned out, I did not have to eat dirt, but I did embark on the most challenging work of my life. Dr. Bredesen developed the road map. I follow it.

I am pleased to have the opportunity to share some of my story with the hope that it will give others the courage to step forward on to the path to reversing their memory loss. I owe my life to Dr. Bredesen, and I will be eternally grateful to him and for the incredible work he has done to bring an end to Alzheimer's for so many people. Bredesen's work sheds light in the dungeon of despair where people with Alzheimer's reside.

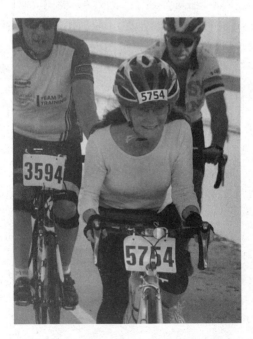

COMMENT: Kristin is now 77 years old, has been following the protocol for nine years, and remains well. Where would we be without Kristin? She was the first, and her diligence and follow-up truly helped to confirm that our theory and conclusions were indeed valid.

When I was asked to see Kristin by her friend, I was worried—we had just been denied in our request to perform a clinical trial of the new protocol we had developed in 2011. We were told by the review committee that the protocol must have only one variable—a drug or a single lifestyle change, not a program. Therefore I had nothing to offer Kristin except the data and conclusions from many years of laboratory experiments. When she called me three months later to tell me how much better she was, I realized that, for the first time, here was an approach that may have the potential to help the many people in need. When I hung up the phone, I turned to my wife and said, "She is better!!"

What if Kristin had given up after a few days? What if she had not been diligent or had ignored most of the program and not realized any benefit? This would have affected many of the subsequent people who would thus not have heard about the program. For no matter how beautiful a theory may sound, data from test tubes, fruit flies, and mice can never replace the need for success in human patients (as T. H. Huxley put it, "The great tragedy of science—the slaying of a beautiful hypothesis by an ugly fact"). Indeed, many proposed Alzheimer's treatments that have proven quite effective in mice have failed in humans. Until Kristin. Therefore, on behalf of all involved—the many patients who have benefited from the protocol, their children and subsequent generations, and all of the physicians, neuropsychologists, nurses, nutritionists, health coaches, and other professionals who have utilized it—my sincere thanks go out to Kristin.

CHAPTER 2

Deborah's Story:
My Father's Daughter

A father holds his daughter's hand for a short while,
but he holds her heart forever.

—ANONYMOUS

For most of my life, I never truly believed that I would get dementia. I worried about it, sometimes a lot, because dementia runs in my family. But somehow I just didn't think it could *actually* happen to me. I was wrong.

My name is Deborah. I am 55 years old. I am married to the love of my life (since college) for the past twenty-nine years. We have four wonderful children, who are now in their teens and 20s, along with a menagerie of dogs and cats. I attended college at Harvard University, graduating with high honors in East Asian studies and government. A few years later, I graduated with honors from the University of Pennsylvania Law School. My professional work has taken me from journalism (ABC News) to law (family law: divorces, child custody) to the theater (acting, directing, and producing, most recently off Broadway).

I tell you all of this because for my story, it matters. It matters because when I was in my 40s, despite all the years of learning how to think, I stopped being able to do it well. I was in the early stages of cognitive decline, on my way toward Alzheimer's dementia. That meant that I could no longer be the kind of mother to my children that I wanted to be, and that working as a journalist or lawyer or theater director no longer seemed like viable professional options for me.

I have thought a lot about how to share my story of having early cognitive decline. When speaking about what happened—to anyone other than my closest friends and family—I have always used a pseudonym or only my first name. Why? Well, in the beginning, I felt embarrassed. And sometimes ashamed. I worried about what people who knew me would think. Would they think I was less intelligent? Would they awkwardly avoid me? Or would they just quietly second-guess me when I gave an opinion? If I lost my keys or forgot what I wanted to say, would they look at me with pity, their eyes saying, *Oh no, she's really going downhill now*? Probably.

I am also hesitant to speak about what happened because on a few occasions when I did dare to open up, I found a few people (although certainly not most) skeptical and dismissive. Was I just "needlessly worrying" about "normal aging"? they'd ask. Or maybe I was just overreacting, they'd suggest with a hint of condescension. I mean, now and again, everyone forgets something, or doesn't recognize someone, or can't find their way, or mixes up words, or can't remember what they've read . . . don't they?

But now, six years after reversing my symptoms by following the Bredesen Protocol, I am as sharp and clear as ever. Every single symptom I had of cognitive decline has disappeared. So I have decided that the time has come for me to tell the full story about what happened to me, openly and honestly, and about how I got better. Everyone should know that Alzheimer's dementia is not only preventable but also, especially in the early stages, reversible. So for all the people out there who might be just like me but not yet realize it, this—my story—is for you.

Seven years ago, I was pretty much in the dark about how dementia starts. I had never heard the words *early cognitive decline.* I didn't know there were initial symptoms that would eventually lead to Alzheimer's. I had no idea that a person could have these symptoms twenty to thirty years before being so impaired that he or she goes to the doctor and gets a diagnosis of Alzheimer's. But I should have.

My grandmother—my father's mother—died from Alzheimer's. She had been a math and physics teacher long before it was common for women to teach those subjects. But when she was in her late 60s, shortly after my grandfather died, she became very confused and forgetful. And then one night, my father got the phone call he had been dreading. The police had found my gentle grandmother wandering a busy Minnesota freeway in the middle of a blizzard. She said she was just heading home to Buffalo, New York, but my father knew otherwise; she was heading toward, in his words, "a living hell."

My father also died from Alzheimer's. Six months ago.

The painful irony of my father's illness and agonizing death escaped no one who knew him. My father was a brilliant and exceptionally compassionate neurologist. He was the doctor that all the specialists would send their "mystery" cases to, because he thought both logically and out of the box. He developed treatments for MS (multiple sclerosis) and pioneered stroke prevention. He found novel ways to alleviate pain, especially for those with migraines, because, he would say, no one should have to suffer. My father often told me, "I'm never allowed to retire," because too many people needed his help. He believed that you must do everything in your power to help another and must never give up. But sometimes there were those whom he couldn't help at all, like those to whom he had to give a diagnosis of Alzheimer's. For those patients, he just sat in our living room and wept.

I always said that I could never give a speech at a memorial for my father because no words could do him justice. And I feel the same writing about him now. So instead I will just say this. Despite all he did for his patients, my father was always there for me, too. When I was older and no longer lived at home, I could call him with any question, big or small, at any time of day or night, and he was immediately present, offering me his gentle guidance. There was no greater giver of wisdom about how I should raise my kids or handle any crisis than my father. He could, I am quite sure, also read my mind, and he always understood exactly how I was feeling without my saying a word. And of all the things we shared, it was our love of dogs that completely bonded us. He gave me my first puppy, Bruno, when I was 23, born to his dog in the kitchen. He nurtured Bruno for the first eight weeks of his life with oatmeal, milk, and honey, and then put him in my arms. "Love," he told me, "is what it's all about."

I do not know when my father realized he had dementia, because we never talked about it. But I do know that he knew. One day, when his memory had started to fail, he got lost while driving his car—very, very lost. He had gone to the supermarket but hadn't returned after many hours. With my daughter by my side, I drove everywhere, desperate to find him. I remember that it was rush hour, and the streets were full of cars and people. Then, as I drove through an intersection about twenty minutes from his house, I saw my father drive past me in a daze. Frantically making a U-turn in the middle of the traffic, I pulled up alongside him, honking to get his attention. He finally looked out his window, saw me, and gave me a little smile. I gestured for him to follow me home, which he did. When we got inside, we sat in the kitchen together, quietly. I explained what had just happened and told him that if he had just found me lost like that, he'd take me to get some "pictures of my brain." He looked at me and with clarity and decisiveness told me, "What I have is something that no one can do anything about." He knew.

But what I don't know is, when exactly did he first recognize his own cognitive decline? Was it only when he started getting lost? Or decades earlier, when he could no longer recognize people's faces well, or when he began to lose his love of reading? I can say from my own experience that it is extremely difficult to recognize the first symptoms of cognitive decline. This is because they can be very subtle, coming on in such small increments that you hardly notice them. One day you might be really good at something, like speaking a foreign language or navigating yourself around a new town, and then years later, you might notice that you aren't actually so good at that anymore. You just don't know why.

For me, my first identifiable symptom of cognitive decline was my struggle to recognize faces. This started around the time I turned 40. I was fine recognizing the people closest to me, but recognizing people one step removed from my immediate circle became problematic. My problem was different from having difficulty remembering someone's name or from not being able to place how or where you've met someone. I just plain couldn't recognize many people I saw on a regular basis. I didn't even have the flicker of recognition you might have when you feel you've met someone but just can't place them. I felt nothing.

I learned to use tricks to identify people. One woman whom I saw often at my children's school, for example, distinguished herself by her especially long black hair, so I could always recognize her as long as she never cut her hair. Other people I came to know by the dog they walked or the bag they carried or perhaps the car they drove. My husband and kids, and my very closest friends, learned to help me out. When people I should know would approach, they would quickly whisper their names to me so I would know who they were.

I will never forget the moment I knew facial recognition was a real issue for me. Working in the baked goods booth at the town fair one summer, I saw people I had met in other contexts coming up to me to buy cakes and cookies. Recognizing me, some tried to start a conversation or ask me questions. But unable to employ my memory tricks (no dog! no bag! no car!), I was lost. Everyone seemed like a stranger to me. I panicked and busied myself for the rest of the day with organizing cakes in the back of the booth.

Toward the end of the day, I took a walk around the fair. I saw a woman holding the hand of her child, waiting for cotton candy. I didn't actually recognize her, but I thought—based upon the hair color and height of each of them—that the mother and child could be the pair I saw usually by the flagpole at school pickup. I said to myself, *You're just insecure. Stop it. Be confident. Take a risk.* So I did. "Hello! How are you?" I asked warmly. She looked at me, startled. "Oh, I'm so sorry," I muttered, and walked away. We didn't know each other at all.

After that, I started to withdraw from certain social situations. I have always wondered if during that time people thought

I was rude or just reclusive. I didn't mean to be either. But it is really frightening not to know who someone is that you are supposed to know; not to know what to say or what to ask. Countless times, I thought I should say, "'I'm so sorry. I have a facial recognition problem. Who are you again?" But I couldn't bring myself to say that. I felt way too embarrassed. When approached by someone who clearly knew me, but whom I didn't recognize, I would (if I could) act like I was in a rush, saying something like, "I'm so sorry, but I'm late picking up my son." Or in the supermarket, I might say, "Oops," as I'd back away from the friendly person, "I forgot apples/ham/cereal [whatever I could think of]," and I'd be off.

At the time, I had no idea that facial recognition difficulties could be one symptom of cognitive decline. Had I known, I might have been more alarmed. Instead, I did some research and decided I had developed prosopagnosia, a more self-limited condition, although not necessarily indicative of a greater problem. I remember asking my father, when he was already in the early stages of Alzheimer's, if he had this problem. He said to me, "Oh yes, if I'm at an event without name tags, I'm lost. I hated those cocktail parties. And doctors' lounges. Much better to just stay home." He had never complained about not recognizing people; he had just withdrawn from situations that might be embarrassing. I concluded (albeit wrongly) that we both had prosopagnosia.

As my 40s progressed, I noticed I wasn't so good at a lot of things I used to be really good at. I had learned several foreign languages in my teens and 20s, but could no longer speak them as I had. My Spanish, in which I had been nearly fluent, had become halting and rusty. My Russian and Chinese, which were both conversant and flowing, seemed to have completely vanished from my brain. On the few occasions when I had an opportunity to speak either one, I couldn't get past hello.

I had also been really good at navigating around new places. When my husband and I would be driving somewhere new, he was the one to ask for directions. I loved the thrill of finding my way without asking anyone. But then things changed. At some point in my 40s, I no longer liked finding my way. I wasn't any good at it anymore. Unknown towns felt like tangled noodles of streets I couldn't separate, and without the navigator, I was in trouble. And driving itself became increasingly anxiety-provoking. It felt like I couldn't control all of the things that could go wrong on any given trip.

And then there was music. I had learned piano as a child, and especially loved to sight-read Broadway show tunes I could sing along to or to play soulful classical music. But somewhere in my 40s, I realized I couldn't really sing anymore. And then, late in my 40s, sitting at a piano for the first time in more than a decade, I looked at a piece of sheet music and realized I couldn't read the notes.

The other cognitive changes I experienced during my 40s were numerous, although none individually seemed especially dramatic, and all could be explained away by thinking I was "just getting older." I started to lose my love of reading because I couldn't always remember what I had read. I dropped out of a course I was taking because I found the material too dense, and I couldn't retain what I had learned, something that had been so easy when I was in college. I found it more and more difficult to participate in meetings, especially those held late in the day. If I had something I wanted to say during one of those meetings, I would often repeat it over and over and over in my head until it was my turn to speak, so that I wouldn't forget what it was.

I also started to tune out of conversations that were not "in my field" because they were hard to understand. I couldn't follow complex movies anymore and would sometimes stay home when my husband and teenage kids would go to the cinema. Remembering to-dos became nearly impossible. My kids learned to write anything they wanted me to remember to do for them on a big piece of paper in the kitchen. They knew that if they didn't do that, it wouldn't get done. I told them it was just so hard to remember things because there was "too much going on." This was especially strange for me, though, because I had always had such a good memory for the little stuff: dates and times; addresses and phone numbers; appointments and lists.

Helping my kids with homework during those years became an increasingly frustrating task, too. I often felt fuzzy when I was trying to understand an assignment or edit their writing. I didn't have access to the same vocabulary I used to have, and felt disheartened I could no longer write with ease. My typing speed plummeted. I had been so fast when I was a lawyer, but then in my 40s, I found my fingers could no longer fly across the keys. I sometimes even had trouble remembering the codes to my gym lockers.

I also started missing, or almost missing, appointments—something I had rarely, if ever, done before. I rationalized that I was just a *very* busy person. But as a result, I became increasingly anxious about keeping track of my schedule, relying more and more on various calendars and alarms to keep me on top of things. During these years, I developed difficulty sleeping and found it frustrating that coffee no longer seemed to help me become alert in the mornings.

Especially troubling for me back then was that I felt mentally exhausted every day after four P.M., for no apparent reason. I wondered why my brain felt so tired. I kept thinking, *What is wrong with me?* But I had no answer.

You might think a lightbulb should have gone off in my head at some point with all my facial recognition problems, or inability to speak foreign languages that I had once been fluent in, or brain fatigue late in the afternoons, that I could be getting dementia. But it didn't. First of all, I didn't know it could come on so young. And second of all, I didn't know what the symptoms were. I just assumed I was getting older, albeit far faster than my friends. I figured I had become rusty at languages and music from lack of practice. Maybe I was in denial. Denial can be a powerful response to a problem that (as far as I knew then) had no solution.

Moreover, each of the cognitive changes I describe above came on with micro-steps over a period of about ten years. To me, this is what makes the onset of Alzheimer's especially insidious. You can't see the progression of the disease when it is happening to you. To make matters worse, a fuzzy brain isn't very good at identifying its weaknesses, so it is unlikely to sound any alarm bells. I can identify all of these changes now only because I have reversed course and have a newfound clarity about what mental skills and cognitive functions had been declining. If I hadn't reversed, I could never have written about any of this.

I remember during that time listening in my car to an interview on NPR one day, and marveling at the journalist's and guest's ability to banter back and forth with seeming ease. How did they do that? Had I once been able to do that, too? What had happened to me? It felt like there was a wall or a cobweb between my brain and the outside world, and it took so much effort to punch through it just to ask a question or make a point, let alone have a meaningful discussion. What used to be easy and fun—engaging in thoughtful dialogue—had become work. Tiring mental work.

More than anything else during those years, though, I just wanted to be a good mother to my children. And I am grateful that at least during that time I could still hug them and love them. I could still pick them up from school and ask about their days. I could still lie with each of them before they went to sleep and talk about their feelings. But I couldn't remember what they wanted from the supermarket. I couldn't keep track of all of their schedules. I couldn't help much with their homework. And I felt like I was struggling to keep up with our lives, unable to really enjoy being together as a result.

People often ask me whether, during those years, my husband was worried. What did he notice? And the answer is that he, like me, knew that some things about me weren't "right," but he didn't know why. He knew I had increasing trouble recognizing people and would try to help me out in social situations, but he didn't know what was causing the problem. He noticed that I was becoming forgetful, sometimes even missing appointments (something especially unusual for me), but assumed that it was because we had so much "going on" in our lives. He observed that I was mentally tired out a lot, especially in the late afternoons and evenings, but thought that this must be what aging looks like. When I told him I felt like my thinking was sometimes fuzzy or that I no longer felt mentally sharp, he'd reassure me that I was too young to be getting dementia. Now, looking back, he talks about how during those years I had become slower in my thinking and that I was using fewer sophisticated words, but that at the time such changes were hard to identify because they were happening so gradually.

To be fair, I had also become pretty good at compensating for what wasn't working so well. My father had been, too, in his 40s and 50s, when he had started to decline. We both found work-arounds for our weaknesses, and we both always did our best to keep up despite slowing down. Neither one of us wanted anyone to know that we weren't as sharp as we had been. As a result, those around me often had no idea how hard I was working just to seem "normal." I was—during those years—kind of like a duck. Watching me swim across the lake, you might have thought I was doing just fine. But if you had looked under the surface, you would have seen that I was paddling like crazy.

And then, when I was almost 48 years old, two things happened that finally made me think I just might be in trouble. One evening, I yelled for my dog in the backyard, but instead of calling her name—"Maisy!"—I called out loudly the dish I was making for dinner—"Chili!" Shortly after that, while driving my kids to school, I announced with confidence to the tollbooth operator that I was a "conference call" to get my discount, rather than a "car pool." These may seem like little word slipups, and maybe they were, but I knew better than to disregard them. I had never made these kinds of mistakes before.

Watching the five o'clock local news some weeks before, my mother had seen a story about a clinic promoting dementia prevention. "Maybe you should check it out," she had gently suggested. "No," I said, "not yet. Maybe in a decade," I had replied. But after years of quiet worrying about my "mental aging," I found those two word slipups set off my personal fire alarm. I needed help. I picked up the phone and called the dementia clinic.

I arrived at my appointment hoping to learn whatever there was known about dementia prevention, and a little scared of what the doctor might find. Sitting in the waiting room with my mother, I saw patients at varying stages of Alzheimer's disease. I felt young and out of place, and was determined to prove that my brain was just fine. In the initial interview, I mentioned a few concerns: my facial recognition problems, feeling "fuzzy" during work meetings, and being so "tired out" much of the time. The doctor then asked me to take a lengthy (several hour) cognitive test. I thought it would be a breeze, but realized after only the first question that the test was actually kind of hard. "What floor are we on?" asked the medical student administering my test. I couldn't remember whether we had taken an elevator or gone up some stairs. I guessed. First floor?

In the end, my results were uneven. Many of my scores were consistent with where they thought I should perform based upon the IQ portion of the test (which, they explained, usually stays fairly intact until the disease is quite progressed). On other parts of the test, though, especially those that were a bit more sophisticated, such as the coding section, I scored far below what was expected, but nothing low enough to cause immediate alarm (below average, for example, but not 10th percentile). The doctor said that since he couldn't say whether my uneven testing represented "normal" for me, we ought to consider this test to be my baseline, and that every six months I could repeat it and see whether there had been a change.

The doctor then recommended that I take a genetic test to see if I carried the common Alzheimer's gene, ApoE4. I initially declined. To me, it seemed there was no point in knowing whether I had the gene when there was nothing significant I could do to prevent it. All he could recommend to me at the time was that I exercise every day, and that I eat, or refrain from eating, certain foods, both of which might, at best, delay (by months? by years?) the onset of Alzheimer's. Why should I get more anxious about my future than I already was?

But I did change my mind and eventually got the genetic test. What finally convinced me was this: the doctor told me that if he knew my genetic status, he might be better able to get me into an Alzheimer's drug trial, should I need that somewhere down the road.

The result shouldn't have surprised me. Given my family history and symptoms, I should have known I would be ApoE4-positive. But when the doctor told me, I was actually shocked and terrified—terrified because I knew exactly what lay ahead for me.

My father had started to change in his 40s, too. He had noticeably "slowed down" over a period of twenty years. He stopped using those fancy words and made up fewer puns and jokes. Somewhere along the way, he lost his love of reading. He stopped writing medical articles. He also became mentally fatigued later in the day, changing his work schedule so that he could leave the hospital by early afternoon. What a contrast that was to the father I grew up with, who routinely worked fourteen- to sixteen-hour days. His social world became narrower, too, and the subjects he liked to talk about became fewer and fewer. And then there was his driving. It became anxiety-provoking. He started to drive exclusively in the slow lane, while the other drivers zipped by. Getting around in new places became an enormous challenge, too.

I am almost certain that at some point during those years, he realized that something was happening to him. But he chose to keep his terror to himself. That was how he was; he wouldn't have wanted to worry anyone. Meanwhile, for the longest time, we—his family—didn't know. We thought he was just exhausted, paying the price for having worked so hard for so many years.

Then, at the age of 67, my father, the man who had always said he'd care for his patients until he turned 100, decided that the time had come for him to close down his medical practice and move down the street from me. "It will be better for your mother that way," he explained.

By then, though, we didn't need to ask why.

Sixty-seven.

I told only a few people about my genetic test. Unlike other diseases, Alzheimer's is not one many people want to talk about. It is terribly stigmatizing, and I especially feared that people would question my capabilities or judgment if they knew. What would this mean for my professional future? But I did confide in my dear friend and sister-in-law, who had written a book on radical remissions from cancer. She was very knowledgeable about new ways to treat disease. She said she had recently come across a paper by Dr. Dale Bredesen called "Reversal of Cognitive Decline," about a protocol followed by ten people with cognitive decline and/or Alzheimer's, nine of whom had reversed. She sent it to me, and for the first time, I had hope.

Determined to delay what I assumed was the inevitable onset of dementia—the best I thought I could hope for—I decided to follow, as best I could, the recommendations Dr. Bredesen made to the initial cohort of patients. I figured I had nothing to lose, and if the protocol bought me any time at all with my husband and children, it would be worth it. Also, Dr. Bredesen wrote in that paper that each person had been "really good" but not "perfect" at following the protocol. That was motivating for me. I remember thinking, *Not perfect, but really good . . . I can do that.*

And so, from one day to the next, I did the following:

I switched to a Mediterranean-style diet, following the principles of the MIND diet I found online (which is similar, although created for those with dementia). Basically, I cut out all "white" sugars and flours. I gave up processed foods. I sought out foods that were organic. I ate mostly vegetables and fruits (primarily berries), eggs, fish or chicken, and only whole grains. I ate lots of olive oil and enjoyed avocados and nuts.

My initial list of diet principles, based in part on the protocol and in part on my own research, was as follows:

No processed foods
Nothing "white": white flour, white sugars, etc. (simple
    carbohydrates) . . . just whole grains
Leafy greens daily
Other vegetables daily
Berries daily (especially blueberries)
Coffee daily (but stay consistent with the amount)
Nuts and seeds daily
Coconut oil/MCT oil daily (I put it in my coffee and use
    for cooking)
Avocados regularly
1 glass of wine some days, red or white
Dark chocolate is okay
Eggs are okay
Some dairy is okay—plain Greek yogurt, low-fat milk
Limited (very infrequent) red meat
Limited (very infrequent) cheese
Fish/poultry okay—fish at least once per week, especially
    salmon
Eliminate fast foods, pastries, sweets, butter, and cream

Since then, I have improved on the diet, cutting back further on the grains and natural sugars. But this is how I started. I'm definitely not perfect, though I like to think I'd get a sticker for being "really good"! And while I do love ice cream (which I do indulge in from time to time), I love my mind more, so that helps me stay the course.

I learned to fast. I started with twelve hours a day, stopping eating after dinner, and not eating again until at least twelve hours had passed. This was difficult for me at first. I loved my morning latte (with a little sugar) as I drove my kids to school, but I switched to unsweetened black or fruit tea. For the first few months, I was really hungry during the last few hours of the fast, but I did eventually adjust. I also often wanted to cheat at night with a little snack, but I (almost always) didn't let myself. Fasting has since become much easier and is now just a part of my daily routine. Now I fast longer, usually thirteen or fourteen hours. That means I try to stop eating a few hours before bed, and don't eat again until thirteen or fourteen hours have passed.

I started to exercise almost every day, between thirty and sixty minutes. If it was only thirty minutes, I made sure it was vigorous. Some exercise had always been a part of my life, but not in a consistent way. I googled for information about exercise and ApoE4, and found a study that showed that those with ApoE4 who exercised vigorously for at least thirty minutes a day, four to six days per week, showed decreases in hippocampal brain volume over many years comparable to those without the gene (regular aging). By contrast, those with the gene who didn't exercise lost brain volume much more precipitously. I had no choice. Vigorous exercise (five or six days per week) was my new job. It was not optional.

I tried to exercise "on my fast." I learned about how my brain, because of the ApoE4, didn't process glucose properly in middle age and beyond, but that ketones—released both by fasting and by exercising—could serve as an alternative food source for my brain. To maximize producing ketones, I tried to exercise before the fast had ended as often as my schedule allowed, at least a few times per week. Sometimes that meant getting up even earlier than I was used to, but I did what I had to do.

I improved on my sleep, as best as I could, trying to get at least seven or eight good hours. I darkened my room and made it cooler. I made sleep a priority, going to bed earlier, often turning in before my children. They in turn learned not to disturb me after I said good night. I started to take melatonin and magnesium before sleep, and L-tryptophan for night awakening.

I introduced supplements into my diet. I started with the "basics," those that Dr. Bredesen recommended to all of those in the initial cohort: fish oil, curcumin, B_{12}, D, probiotics, and alpha-lipoic acid. Then I slowly added in others, one at a time, so I could see what effect they might have on me and adjust accordingly (did they make me sleepy? nauseated?): ashwagandha, *Bacopa monnieri*, citicoline, CoQ10 (ubiquinol), vitamin B complex (on days when I didn't take B_{12}). Later, I would add in pregnenolone, NAC (for insulin resistance), vitamin C, zinc, and manganese, as I learned what I was deficient in, and what might benefit me specifically.

Two years later, I started bioidentical hormones—estrogen and progesterone—to help me with menopausal symptoms and improve my sleep, in addition to the cognitive benefits they might confer. But this is not something I started with, for a variety of reasons personal to me.

Dr. Bredesen also recommended that the initial cohort work on de-stressing and brain stimulation. I did try to be more mindful about what stressed me and to limit those stressors. And I tried (albeit not so successfully) to find time to meditate or breathe calmly. But in the beginning, I couldn't really figure out how to limit stress in a more thoughtful way. As for brain stimulation, I had tried the app called Lumosity, but found it discouragingly hard. The thought of learning a language or an instrument felt overwhelming. What I didn't know at the time was that my brain would improve, and that when it did, the brain stimulation part of the protocol would become the most fun.

I started the protocol in late April 2015. Knowing I had ApoE4, together with watching my father decline, gave me the strength and determination to stick with it. I knew my life depended on it. That said, I had absolutely no expectation of experiencing improvements. As a result, when the improvements came (which they did with a vengeance), I was completely taken by surprise.

Fast-forward three months, to July. In the middle of an exercise class one day, I looked around and suddenly realized that I actually recognized some people. Even more, I *knew* that I knew them. I had never had that feeling in that class before. In fact, I usually felt embarrassed to say hello to others because I was never certain that I knew them.

Fast-forward another two months, to September. I attended Parents' Day at my kids' school. That day was typically anxiety-provoking for me because I wasn't sure who people were or whether I *should* know them (unless they put on a name tag). This time, though, I actually had fun. Not only did I recognize people, but I knew that I knew them and enjoyed going up to people and engaging in conversation.

Fast-forward another month, to October. My True Awakening. Over a period of four to six weeks, other changes came on, one after another. Literally from one day to the next, it felt like I was waking up further, like a fog was lifting from my brain. I began to feel mentally much sharper. I became much more alert in meetings and in conversations. My reading comprehension and recollection greatly improved. I suddenly really *wanted* to read again; I *wanted* to learn. Then one day I noticed that I was using much more sophisticated words to explain what I meant: petulant instead of grouchy; fastidious instead of picky; pugnacious instead of aggressive.

Also during that time, my "four o'clock fatigue" dissipated. Prior to that, I had dreaded the time from four to ten P.M., when my kids needed me most but when my mind was just too tired. Suddenly (and it truly felt sudden) I was mentally alert up until bedtime. Homework help? No problem! Late-night run to the supermarket? Sure! I realized then that the "four o'clock fatigue" had come on so slowly, so insidiously, that I hadn't recognized it for what it was: the creeping in of dementia.

My memory started to improve then, too. I no longer needed my kids to leave me those reminder notes on big pieces of paper in the kitchen. I kept track of my schedule again, often in my head. Likewise, I felt more in control and confident when driving. A calm set in. I began to enjoy lengthy, complex conversations and complicated movies. I even noticed that when I drank coffee in the mornings, I actually felt the caffeine effect again.

One day around that time, I sat down to write something and noticed two things. One, I could type really fast. Suddenly my fingers were flying across the keyboard just as they had twenty years earlier. And two, I found that I actually could *write*. I had ideas. And they were flowing.

That was when I knew I was back.

Shortly thereafter, in early December, I repeated the several-hour battery of cognitive tests. The low scores from my first test had jumped from average or below average to the top percentiles.

The neurologist who administered the test told me that, given the dramatic improvement, he could say that while previously I'd been in early cognitive decline, I had definitely fully resolved.

There is not a day that goes by since I sat in that doctor's office that I do not think of my gratitude toward Dr. Bredesen. His protocol saved my life. How can you properly thank someone for that?

I have since stayed true to the protocol, and plan to do so for the rest of my life. When my schedule (travel, illness) has interfered somewhat with the protocol, I have noticed some backsliding into fuzzy thinking. But redoubling my efforts each time has brought me back to where I was.

Following the program isn't always easy. It requires being deliberate, consistent, and determined about each aspect. It requires self-acceptance of imperfection, because I don't think anyone can follow it perfectly, all the time. I also think it helps to start as soon as you can. Because I was just in the very early stages of decline, I had a relatively easy time adjusting my habits and changing my lifestyle. Finally, I think that being successful on the protocol takes finding loving support, whether it be from a spouse or family member or friend. I am blessed to have a beautiful husband who has cheered me on from the first day. He exercises with me and encourages me to stay the course with the diet and the fast, and to get my sleep. I am grateful to him every single day.

Since the initial "awakening," I have also experienced other improvements in my cognitive functioning, some of which are subtle but still significant to me. I have no doubt that I am back to my old self in my meetings and discussions. Complex books and movies (I loved *Bridge of Spies!*) are pleasurable now. Carrying on conversations is no longer "work," and I definitely don't need to repeat what I want to say in my head anymore for fear of forgetting. I feel sharp and analytical again.

My facial recognition problem remains a thing of the past. My spoken Spanish returned to where it had been, and some of the Chinese and Russian I had learned remarkably came back, too, sometimes in waves of words. I am also really good at navigating myself around new places again. No longer tangles of noodles, new places are like puzzles for me to piece together. And I definitely can remember all of my to-dos, dates, and appointments. I used to be so panicked that I would forget something—a pickup from school, a doctor's appointment, a flight even—but that stress is gone.

It was about a week into following the protocol when I discovered I couldn't read music anymore. After two years on the protocol, however, I sat down again at a piano. Curious, I put up a piece of music, and as if by magic, all the notes made sense to me. It is hard to describe how incredible it feels to look at music that had been impossible to read and find it suddenly, completely legible, without having put in a minute's work to relearn it. Now playing the piano serves as de-stressing and brain stimulation all rolled into one.

On reflection, I can now see that what I, and my father before me, faced midlife were clear early symptoms of dementia: increasing facial "blindness"; "four o'clock fatigue"; anxiety about schedules and appointments (and sometimes missing them); a gradual loss of interest in reading, movies, and complex conversations; gradually decreasing clarity and thinking speed; a gradual decrease in vocabulary; intermittent word-search problems; slipups with language; anxiety about driving and difficulty navigating; difficulty remembering to-dos; a loss of foreign language and musical skills; and sleep disruption. There was a pattern there. I just hadn't seen it.

Reversing my decline taught me that so much of what I had learned, whether it be languages or music or vocabulary, was actually still in my brain. I just couldn't access the information. I hadn't lost the ability to read music or speak foreign languages. I hadn't forgotten sophisticated vocabulary. I just couldn't access the part of my brain where those skills, and those words, were coded in. Other skills, like facial recognition or navigation, short-term memory or thinking fast, came back effortlessly, as if I had just been lacking the necessary cognitive fuel.

I often sat next to my father when he was in the late stages of Alzheimer's, holding his hand, and wondered what was still inside of his brain. Had his words and memories actually all disappeared? Or could he just not access them, like me?

About two years before he died, my father could no longer recognize me. He forgot he had a daughter, and he didn't know my name. But he often cried when he saw me, and he always told me he loved me. I couldn't help wondering what it meant that his cognitive pathways seemed impassable but that his emotional pathways still worked. Did this enable him to access the part of his brain where his memories were stored, eliciting an emotional, though not a cognitive, response? Then, days before his death, and reduced to a working vocabulary of only a few words, my father saw a poster on the wall and called out, "That's Einstein!" And indeed it was. Somehow, in the dramatic denouement of his life, my father found the fuel to access his memory of a man named Einstein.

Anyone who has witnessed Alzheimer's knows this: the cruelty of the disease is extreme, from the terrifying mental crumbling to the physical devastation that follows. It can last for years upon years upon years. The suffering my father endured is beyond words, beyond explanation, and it haunts me every single day. In the end, all my father wanted was to get back to Buffalo, like his mother had, to get away from the pain. If only that would have helped.

No one should ever have to suffer as my father did. No one.

I do know my father would have been relieved to know that, finally, the cycle of Alzheimer's in our family has been broken. He would have been so happy to know that I can follow a protocol that prevents, and even reverses, the disease, and that his grandchildren will be able to as well. He always cared more about others than he did about himself, and this was true even until his very end. But oh, how I wish he could have followed it, too.

I know something else. My father would have wanted me to share our story, to do what I can to help others. So I owe it to him, and his legacy, to do so. It is the least I can do.

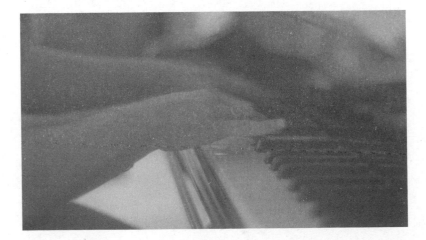

COMMENT: I am grateful to Deborah for sharing her story with all of us. It is at once poignant and triumphant. Her history illustrates several important points, ones common to many patients. First, she noticed very clear cognitive changes in her 40s. Research has shown that the brain changes of Alzheimer's disease, reflected in changes in the spinal fluid and amyloid imaging, begin about twenty years before a diagnosis, so that what we used to think of as a disease of our 60s, 70s, and 80s has turned out to be a disease that does indeed often start in the 40s—and even earlier in some people. Second, not only can the ability to make new memories return, but old, seemingly lost memories can themselves return—in Deborah's case, her ability to play the piano returned, as did her ability to speak foreign languages. Third, Deborah's cognitive ability did not plateau after a few months, but rather continued to improve with time and continued optimization of her personalized protocol.

As heartbreaking as Deborah's story is for her father and grandmother, it is a story of hope for Deborah, her children, and future generations of her family. I look forward to the day when each and every family can be certain that Alzheimer's disease will never again darken its door.

CHAPTER 3

Edward's Story: Outdistancing Alzheimer's

Is this the promised end?

—WILLIAM SHAKESPEARE, *KING LEAR*

What does it feel like to be told that you have Alzheimer's disease? What thoughts rush through your mind, what images of your children and grandchildren, of your life's passions and accomplishments, of your exultations and regrets? You cannot know until you have experienced it.

Alzheimer's—is there a more dreaded word? Even with cancer, there are many examples of survivors, but with Alzheimer's, everything was bleak. It was 2003, and I had just been told that I had early Alzheimer's. But I am getting ahead of myself. My name is Edward, and if you remember me from *The End of Alzheimer's*, then here you'll read my side of the story: I grew up in the Pacific Northwest and went to college on an athletic scholarship. (Fortunately, I did not have any sports-related concussions, but I did once do a face-plant on an ice rink, with a brief loss of consciousness.)

While in college, I became interested in the health professions, and ended up pursuing graduate studies, then setting up my own practice. Things went swimmingly well until in my mid-40s, when something unusual began to happen: I would get exasperated with my staff at times—they often seemed to be on a different page than I was. As I found out only later, when I would be irritated by someone's telling me that they had told me something before, and I'd say, "That's the first I've heard of it," they would furtively roll their eyes. Some of the staff began to complain to my wife, who worked with me, that I often forgot something I had been told. In retrospect, it was a harbinger of what was to come.

These occasional office problems continued into my 50s, but I was still able to do my job very effectively. However, in my late 50s, I traveled to an event in Europe with many relatives and friends, and something had changed: I was stressed, I was jet-lagged, and I simply could not organize the events as I should have been able to do. I could not multitask as I had for years. Something was very wrong, and I called a close friend to ask for help.

When I flew back to the States, I went back to the gym to work out. I stared at my locker and realized that I had no idea what the lock combination was! I had been away for only two weeks—how could I have forgotten the combination to a locker I had used so often? It did not seem to make sense. I racked my brain, but never did come up with the combination, and the lock had to be cut. That is when I knew for certain that something must be wrong.

I realized that I had to be evaluated for my memory lapse, especially since my father had developed dementia, but I was leading a large department and wanted my evaluation to remain anonymous, at least for now. I searched my brain to come up with something benign that might have caused my recent problems. Stress? Depression? Perhaps a metabolic problem like diabetes or episodes of hypoglycemia? I knew that one of my colleagues who was a neurological expert was going to be relocating, so I sought her out for a confidential discussion. I underwent PET scanning under a pseudonym, hoping that the test would show nothing of concern. That's when my world, my future, my hopes, all changed: the PET scan showed a very typical pattern for Alzheimer's disease. My neurological colleague told me that I had early Alzheimer's, and that this was "the beginning of a journey." It was a journey I was very reluctant, even horrified, to take, but one that I knew now was inevitable.

I was referred to a neuropsychologist. Now that I knew what was going on, I wanted to know how much of my cognitive ability I had lost. I actually scored pretty well on this initial testing, so the neuropsychologist said, "Well, maybe the pattern on your PET scan is something you've had your whole life— maybe it doesn't mean Alzheimer's after all." He and I both knew that wasn't the case, but it was helpful and hopeful to hear about anything other than ineluctable decline.

I called my ex-wife, since her parents had both died from Alzheimer's disease and she'd had extensive experience with it. It was frightening to hear the stories. I increased my life insurance. I thought carefully. I worried about my young daughter. I rewrote my will.

I dabbled with thoughts of suicide, but I did not want to leave that burden with my family. I considered a carefully orchestrated "accident" (one that would also preserve the life insurance), but recognized that this was likely to fail. I avoided telling my family what was going on, feeling there was no point, since I knew that there was nothing that could be done. I resolved to continue to work as long as I could.

Over the next couple of years, I noticed that my math skills were deteriorating. I had always been able to make mental calculations very quickly, and that ability disappeared. When my daughter needed help with her math, I hired a tutor, realizing that in the past I could have helped her easily. I struggled to remember how to spell the name of one of my relatives. Mental activity was exhausting. Anything that was rote was preserved, but for anything that involved novelty or reasoning, I struggled.

I tried Aricept (donepezil), but saw no improvement, and I worried that someone would see me with this medication, so I discontinued taking it. I had difficulty solving staffing problems and could not deal with the personality variations from one person to another. I also lost my ability to prioritize—a lightbulb that needed changing seemed just as pressing as a critical personnel problem. I often forgot the person with whom I'd had lunch.

My next neuropsychological testing showed some decline, but to my surprise it was relatively modest, so I hoped that I might avoid rapid deterioration. Unfortunately, however, the follow-up testing showed very significant decline. The neuropsychologist told me that there was no recovery from Alzheimer's, so I should shut down my office. I searched for any sign of optimism or hope from him—the same neuropsychologist who had earlier told me that perhaps my PET scan pattern was developmental rather than degenerative—but it was gone. It was clear that my decline was accelerating and irreversible.

I struggled after the neuropsychologist told me it was time to shut down my work life. What would I do? And why was the decline accelerating?

My ex suggested that I go to the Buck Institute and talk with Dr. Dale Bredesen, but I was skeptical. After all, why would this guy have the answer when no one else did? Was there really something new on the planet? After the almost daily "headlines" we all hear about "breakthroughs" in Alzheimer's, I was indeed skeptical. However, since there wasn't any effective alternative, I thought I might as well at least find out more.

Late in 2013, then, I met with Dale, and we went over the various contributors to cognitive decline that his research team and he had studied over the decades, and the exciting initial results they were seeing by translating these research findings to the clinical setting. Even through my accelerating brain fog, I could understand the idea of "thirty-six holes in the roof," which require more than one patch to address the problem. At the very least, the protocol he described should make me healthier, I thought, so with little downside, why not try it?

I found out that I have a single copy of ApoE4, so I am indeed in a high-risk group for Alzheimer's disease. I found out that my homocysteine was very high at 18, whereas it should be less than 7 for minimizing brain atrophy with age. This suggested that I may not have been getting enough vitamin B_6, folate, and B_{12}. My vitamin D was low at 28, and my pregnenolone was very low at 6, whereas it should be closer to 100. My zinc was low (most of us actually have suboptimal zinc—about a billion people worldwide—especially those taking proton pump inhibitors for acid reflux), my free copper too high, and I had signs of systemic inflammation. I realized that, metabolically speaking, I had lots to fix.

As I looked over the list of the various contributors to cognitive decline—from viral infections to inflammation to insulin resistance to various toxic exposures, and on and on—I realized that I might indeed have contributed to my own cognitive challenges. I was eating a fairly standard American and European diet, low in good fats and high in French fries; I was drinking moderately but probably not the best amount for someone struggling with cognitive issues; I was living a high-stress life with a multi-site thriving business; and I was not getting optimal sleep, among other potentially important factors. On the other hand, I was doing *some* things right, at least: I was exercising most days, and I was taking the antiviral Valtrex. I wondered whether the Valtrex might actually have helped to slow my decline over the first years after diagnosis, even though at the time I did not connect those dots and had been taking the Valtrex simply to suppress the occasional *Herpes* cold sore outbreaks.

In 2013, nothing had yet been published on the results achieved with Dr. Bredesen's protocol, but I resolved to give it a try with some help from my loved ones. Even as I was starting it, however, as a practical person I knew that my expectations should not be too high. Therefore, even as I was starting the protocol, I met with my best friend, both of us in contemplative moods. We agreed that we had both had fantastically good lives, even if mine might be drawing to a close.

Over the next few months, I focused on getting the protocol right: I completely overhauled my diet—out with the fries, out with the alcohol; in with the salads and oils, the nighttime fasting, and the plant-rich ketogenic diet—exercised heavily each day, improved my sleep, reduced my stress, and took a raft of supplements designed to optimize my neurochemistry. Each morning I would swim in cold water or cycle long distances. As I sped along mile after mile, bearing down, faster and faster, I began to wonder— might I actually outdistance Alzheimer's?

The first change was actually a *lack* of change. A family member noted that the cognitive decline, which had been accelerating for about eighteen months before I began the protocol, had completely stopped. That was a welcome development. Then I began to note a return of my cognitive function and a lifting of the fog. The faces at work were more immediately recognizable, my lunch partners were no longer forgotten, and my facility with math began to return. After I had been on the protocol about six months, it was clear that things were on the mend.

Prior to starting the protocol, I had been instructed by the neuropsychologist to close my offices and begin to get my affairs in order, since it was only a matter of time before I would need daily assistance. Now, a year later, after improving, I had a very different decision to make: Should we open a new office as well as keeping the old ones? After careful consideration, I decided that it would be a good idea, and indeed this new office has turned out to be successful.

I found that the protocol, which had been a bit of a bother at first—changing behavior always is—became progressively easier as I inserted it into my daily living. It became second nature. Well, almost. Okay, I still had the occasional French fries and sometimes also some wine. But for the most part, I was living the protocol. And things at work were back to normal—imagine that!

Of course I never knew how long the improvement was going to last, but most of the time I did not think about that, because I was busy with my life once again. I worked, I traveled, I vacationed, I spent time with family and friends; I thrived. And the improvement continued.

After nearly two years, Dale suggested that I undergo repeat quantitative neuropsychological testing in order to document the improvement I had experienced. *Whoa, there's a loaded suggestion,* I thought. What if the neuropsychologist tells me that the "improvement" I've noticed—heck, others have noticed it, as well—is simply not true? What if this is all a placebo effect? Hey, I'm doing great, do I really care if it's a placebo effect? But if it is, I don't want to know. It would crush me to find out that it was all a dream, and it would likely compromise future functioning. Besides, the neuropsychologist had always been somewhat pessimistic (not surprising, of course, given his years of experience with Alzheimer's patients). So, as much as I understood the need to determine the efficacy of the protocol, I did not want to disturb my ongoing routine.

However, I was finally convinced to repeat the testing, since it might ultimately help others to know whether the protocol I—and others like me—had used was proven to be effective or not. So, somewhat reluctantly, I went back for testing in late 2015, about two years after starting the protocol. Just as for the previous testing sessions, I spent several hours as the neuropsychologist probed all aspects of my brain's functioning. I held my breath for the results . . .

To my great relief, the results were excellent! The scores were strikingly improved. In fact, the neuropsychologist pointed out that he had not seen such improvements in patients with Alzheimer's in his many years of practice. Not only did my memory scores improve, but the speed of processing—essentially a measure of how "young" my brain is functioning—improved as well.

So, according to the tests, I actually had a younger-acting brain than I had had in the past.

I have now been on the protocol for over seven years, and the improvement continues to this day. Sure, occasionally I may forget something, but don't we all? I am in my mid-70s now, working and functioning as well as ever. I am grateful that I have been able to watch my daughter grow up to become an accomplished lady, and grateful for the time with my family.

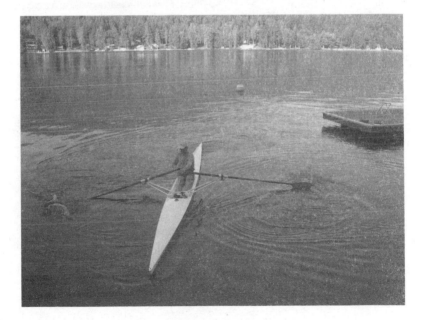

COMMENT: Men represent about a third of Alzheimer's patients, and men who are ApoE4-positive about 20 percent of all Alzheimer's patients. Edward followed a course that is seen commonly: slow decline over a period of several years, followed by accelerating decline. He had his first clear symptoms during a period of great stress, which is another common feature. His genetics showed that he is a member of the high-risk ApoE4-positive group, and his PET scan confirmed his diagnosis of Alzheimer's disease.

What does it feel like to be marching along in a successful career, still relatively young, and be blindsided by the early, and then progressive, symptoms of Alzheimer's disease? Unfortunately, Edward found out. Fortunately, he has experienced a return—a sustained return, now for over seven years—of his excellent cognitive abilities. Since he works helping many in the healthcare profession, his success is actually a story of success for thousands.

CHAPTER 4

Marcy's Story: Disaster Relief

I always tried to turn every disaster into an opportunity.

—JOHN D. ROCKEFELLER

Hi, everyone, my name is Marcy, and I'm a retired psychiatrist who is 79 years old. I graduated from Columbia College of Physicians and Surgeons. I have lived in Westchester, New York, with my significant other for twenty years in a house I built in 1991. I have a lovely daughter and son-in-law who live only an hour away with my three grandchildren. My talented and much-loved son died at age 29 in 2001.

My mother had dementia secondary to hydrocephalus. She died after a fall following shunt surgery that had somewhat improved her dementia. My oldest sister frequently complained of memory problems. She died at age 80 following a ruptured abdominal aneurysm. My other older sister, age 82, also has complained about memory problems. She has frequent falls because she said she cannot remember she is old and should look out for tripping hazards. My younger brother has no memory problems.

I'm very busy all the time with a high-level, complicated volunteer job and several public health and environmental advocacy projects.

Learning disabilities run in my family. I had them in math, spelling, and grammar. As a child, I was tutored in spelling in second grade. In medical school, my disabilities made my studies a struggle, especially in biochemistry and math-related subjects. The same persistence and hard work required to get ahead with learning disabilities have aided my sticking to the many aspects of the Bredesen Protocol.

I had an excellent memory in medical school, training, and practice until I turned 50. I moved to Westchester, New York, in 1991. At the time I was building my own house, living in it while many toxic finishes and paints were being applied. Simultaneously I began to notice my memory was not as good as it had been.

In 2003, unrelated to my memory, I participated in the Mount Sinai/Commonweal Body Burden study of toxics found in the body. I was found to have 31 chemicals affecting the brain and nervous system.

My memory problems concerned me enough while I was visiting the Canyon Ranch in December 2006, that I took an hour-long memory test, the Wechsler Memory Scale, third edition (WMS-III). The results for my age were immediate memory 23rd percentile, and delayed memory 20th percentile. The psychologist doing the test recommended I should seek further testing and help. Fortunately, I forgot this advice, as there was no one able to reverse my type of memory problem until Dr. Bredesen created his protocol.

My main memory symptom was an inability to remember new information, such as names, faces, books, newspapers, movies, plays, lectures, names of frequently visited restaurants, and fact-based conversations. It was as if information was erased as it was strained through my brain. For instance, unless I underlined passages, I could read the same pages over again and again without knowing I had already read them. I was unable to remember the names of the trees and plants on my property, no matter how many times I reviewed the labels.

I could play four hours of golf with someone new and then see him or her a month later but not remember their face or name. Also, I could not recall the names of many people with whom I'd played over the years, even though I knew their faces. It was even hard to remember the number of strokes on each hole, not to mention how to play certain shots. Although I had played golf since age ten and had become quite good, now it was as if I had partly forgotten how to play.

The increasing severity of the memory loss made me avoid some of the activities I had previously enjoyed. Aside from the enjoyment and interest that happened in the moment, no information stuck.

Some of my other memory symptoms caused problems that ranged from expensive to extremely dangerous. One hundred percent of the time I would forget to put money in the parking meter despite a large pile of parking tickets. I would also forget to check myself and the dog for ticks, despite living at the epicenter of the Lyme epidemic and having already contracted two tick-borne diseases, Lyme and ehrlichiosis. I would forget to put on sunscreen despite having had multiple skin cancers. Most dangerous was forgetting to look for pedestrians and bicycles while driving in New York City. I was on the verge of giving up driving. (Now I have become a safe driver again, and I remember to put money in the meter every time.)

Another odd memory symptom was almost complete amnesia

about the personal details of my life, especially my childhood. I could recall the name of only one teacher before medical school and one teacher in medical school. Also, I could remember no details of travel or times playing with siblings, and few memories of specifics about the lives of friends.

I would mention to friends that I had trouble with my memory. One day, one of these friends told me that he had learned about Dr. Bredesen and had read one of his research papers; my friend thought he might be able to help me. I immediately found that paper and saw that some patients who had had a worse memory than mine had gotten better, so I felt there was no reason Dr. Bredesen's protocol would not help me. Being a physician, I ordered the blood tests myself and then took them to a local functional medicine doctor, who prescribed the indicated vitamins and supplements for low thyroid, disturbed levels of estrogen, progesterone, and testosterone, low vitamins D and B12, and other deficiencies.

Following the protocol on my own, on September 9, 2016, I went to NYU Langone's Pearl I. Barlow Center for Memory Evaluation and Treatment and had an MRI and a PET scan, which came back showing signs that might be consistent with early Alzheimer's. My hippocampus was at only the 16th percentile for my age. The NYU neurologist offered me Aricept (a medicine commonly prescribed for Alzheimer's disease), but I declined it. Although it helped early symptoms, I knew it did not alter the course of the disease.

The neurologist was unfamiliar with Dr. Bredesen's work, and therefore was understandably not interested that I was following his protocol.

After this MRI diagnosis on October 20, 2016, I emailed Dr. Bredesen for the first time. I wanted his help because I did not know how to order some of the tests mentioned in his research papers, nor did I know how to interpret the MRI. Fortunately, he responded in a very kind and helpful manner, and began guiding me in many ways, including suggesting tests and explaining their results. Eventually I found that I had thirty-three abnormal blood tests, including Lyme and five heavy metals found in the heavy metal stimulation test. Fortunately, the APOE genetic test for Alzheimer's risk was ApoE 3/3, indicating typical risk rather than the increased risk associated with ApoE4.

Looking back, I am amazed that I was only slightly anxious about the diagnosis of possible early Alzheimer's. The relative lack of anxiety was because Dr. Bredesen said if I followed his protocol closely and continually, I might never get Alzheimer's disease, and I believed him because that was what his research was showing. I could also tell that Dr. Bredesen was an honest and sincere man of enormous intelligence, an encyclopedic knowledge of the brain, and deep dedication.

Following the Bredesen Protocol and the recommendation of the NYU neurologist, I had four hours of neuropsychological testing on November 9, 2016, administered by Elisa Livanos, PhD. Dr. Livanos said in her summary: "Despite the identified significant hippocampal volume loss shown on neuroimaging, the findings of this evaluation are not consistent with what would be expected of an individual with a neurodegenerative disease process (i.e., Alzheimer's disease affecting the temporal lobe structures)."

I was delighted and relieved with these results. They confirmed my own impression of improvement, and indicated to me that the Bredesen Protocol, which I had now been following for about eight months, was working.

I increased my efforts to follow the KetoFLEX 12/3 diet and to get into ketosis. I lost 14 pounds and became almost too thin. I also increased exercise. Then on May 7, 2017, a heavy metal stimulation test with DMSA (a medication that pulls heavy metals out of the bones and brain) was done. It showed that my mercury was extremely elevated, and so were my lead, cesium, arsenic, and thallium.

I'd had a large number of mercury fillings as a child, and these had gradually been replaced with gold inlays. Also, I had lived in an old house, built in 1893, while its lead pipes were being replaced. Despite being worried about chelation (a treatment designed to reduce heavy metals), in time I decided to do it. I hoped to lower the high mercury and lead, which could be playing a major role in my memory problems.

Around this time, when blood tests indicated that I had Lyme and possibly mold-produced mycotoxins, Dr. Bredesen referred me to Dr. Mary Kay Ross, a practicing internist then in Savannah, Georgia, who is an expert in the Bredesen Protocol and the treatment of Lyme, mold, and toxins. I first saw her on February 16, 2017.

On April 2, 2018, the Great Plains Lab test for toxic non-metals was done and revealed high levels of four toxins: those found in dry cleaning, nail polish, flame retardants, and organophosphate pesticides. Even though I do not use pesticides on my property, I have been exposed on golf courses for years. Since getting those results, I have stopped using nail polish and hair dye and have found a "greener" cleaner that does not use "perc" (perchloroethylene), a dangerous respiratory irritant, neurotoxin (which has been associated with Parkinson's disease), and possible carcinogen. I also use the least toxic cleaning and personal care products.

Before I could start chelation on July 3, 2018, I was admitted to the hospital because of a fever of 102.8, extreme exhaustion, and very low platelets and low white blood cells, which resulted in the diagnosis of ehrlichiosis, a tick-borne disease. I had twenty-four hours of treatment with IV doxycycline and Zosyn, followed by two weeks of oral doxycycline. This treatment was doubly fortunate, since it seemed to have immediately gotten rid of the ehrlichiosis and also gotten rid of some lingering Lyme, so *finally* I had the energy to do more of the kind of aerobic exercise that had played such a central role in the healing of Dr. Bredesen's other patients.

After my liver enzymes had recovered from the ehrlichiosis and I had done many courses of IV glutathione (which is critical for detoxification) to correct an abnormally low level, I was ready to start chelation for the high levels of mercury and lead previously revealed in the 500 mg DMSA pretest.

After two rounds of chelation, my mercury levels dramatically decreased from a high of 27 mcg/g in the pre-chelation test to a normal of 2.4. Lead decreased from 18 in the pre-chelation test to 5.7 (the normal for lead is below 2). Many other heavy metals decreased, and aluminum was virtually gone. My excellent practitioner, Sallie Minniefield, PA, at the Schachter Center for Complementary Medicine in Suffern, New York (now sadly closed), said it was the best result she had seen in twenty-five years of doing chelation.

METHOD OF CHELATION

I took 100 mg DMSA three days in a row, then skipped a week and did five cycles and retested. On the fourth chelation of the first round, I got clear symptoms of new information being forgotten at an alarmingly high rate, and decreased the DMSA dose to 50 mg for the fifth and final chelation. (The information draining through my mind alarmingly fast from too much DMSA confirmed that my main symptom of new information draining through my brain too fast was somehow connected with too much mercury or lead having been pulled into my blood by the chelation.)

On October 12, 2018, the MRI and the follow-up PET scan showed that "No specific atrophy or hypometabolism is present to suggest a neurodegenerative process." The neurologist was extremely impressed that the signs of neurodegeneration had disappeared. I was ecstatic. I brought the same neurologist a copy of Dr. Bredesen's book, and he was so happy and interested to receive it that he thanked me three times.

On September 3, 2019, I took a 500 mg DMSA, and six hours later tested to see if my post-chelation levels had stayed stable, but unfortunately I found that my lead levels were up to 7.9 and mercury to 8.9, also significantly increased, meaning further chelation would be indicated if I thought the risk-reward ratio made it worth doing.

In November of 2019 I was extremely encouraged and happy to get the great news that the volume of my brain's hippocampus— a critical area for memory formation, and the area often most heavily affected in Alzheimer's—had dramatically increased since 2016: from 54 percent and then 50 percent in 2017 to 60 percent in 2019. Dr. Cyrus Raji, a neuroradiologist, read all three scans using a computer-based program called Neuroreader.

In November 2019, I went to Seattle to see Dr. Ross and meet her excellent Brain Health and Research Institute team. They have all been very helpful, especially Dr. Ross; the health coach, Kerry Mills; and the physical trainer, Corwin Patis. Corwin has the unique approach of training the mind at the same time as the body.

Finally, in May of 2020, I was diagnosed by a home sleep study with mild sleep apnea. The AHI (apnea-hypopnea index) tells you how many times you stop breathing each hour, and it should be less than 5. Unfortunately, mine was 10.5, but after two months on CPAP treatment, it is back to a normal of 1 or sometimes 2. The sleep study was suggested by Dr. Bredesen, since sleep apnea is a common contributor to memory problems and reduced brain volume in the hippocampus. I have the DreamMapper app connected to my Philips CPAP machine, so every morning I can see the number of apneas (when I stop breathing) and hypopneas (when I slow my breathing too much) that occurred that previous night. Also helpful is Naväge, a relatively easy and quick form of nasal irrigation that relieves the nasal congestion from allergies that contributes to my sleep apnea.

When I have tried to tell friends about my memory problems (except for my closest family and friends), people have either not accepted that I had a serious memory problem or not accepted the possibility that it was permanently gone, despite the many ways it had impacted my life. Both of these reactions made me anxious, threatening the confidence and hope I needed to do the daily work on the program. Support from Dr. Bredesen and Dr. Ross has been essential for my continued improvement. It has mostly offset my not being able to share my daily struggles of having a severe memory problem and adhering to the protocol. The help of a few friends and a supportive significant other has also been essential.

In addition to the KetoFLEX 12/3 diet, exercise, the supplements, chelation, the Lyme and ehrlichiosis treatment, and the use of the CPAP machine, the single thing that has helped me the most is the brain training from BrainHQ. For over three years I have played every morning, an average of 40 minutes per day, with fewer than five missed days. I also follow my percent of progress and stage and level of each game closely to be sure I'm not going backward. The diversity of the games helps keep me from being bored. I force myself to stop playing after 40 minutes and go out and do aerobics now that my energy is back because the Lyme disease is gone.

When I started playing BrainHQ, I was in the 20th percentile for my age, but now I'm in the 89th percentile for someone age 79.

Dr. Bredesen explained that BrainHQ has decades of brain research behind it, and I am sure it helps wake up my brain synapses every morning. I am also sure that playing the games has improved my driving, so that I am a good driver once again. I also think it has played an important role in the increase in the size of my hippocampus and in my overall improved memory.

I have also been helped by the game Elevate, which is very different but helpful for daily life. When I first started playing, I failed the name recall game over 100 times before I passed. Now I'm in the 93.7th percentile. Repeating failing games illustrates the type of persistence I needed to make real improvement.

In the last year I have started playing online CodyCross, an easy and non-frustrating crossword puzzle game. Also I started Boggle online with my grandchildren, ages 6 and 8. They beat me all the time and have much faster brain speeds, but I'm improving bit by bit and having fun, especially during COVID, when it's so much harder to see them.

Now I'm very fortunate that my daily life is not impacted by memory issues. I'm extremely alert, focused, and sharper, and I can recall what people told me weeks earlier. I can do my volunteer job more effectively. My golf game has returned, and I can remember my number of strokes and how to play specialty shots better. My significant other, who previously described my memory as "disastrous," later said it had improved to where it was "just plain lousy." Now he says I "have a mind like a steel trap"—quite an improvement from when I started!

Some information is still erased as it "drains" through my brain, but much less, and I'm hopeful that continuing all the parts of the protocol and getting into ketosis and lowering my still-high mercury and lead levels will improve that problem. But if I never get any better, I can happily live out my life having walked away from the edge of Alzheimer's disease.

Naturally, I will be endlessly grateful to Dr. Bredesen for his amazingly effective program, which saved my mind.

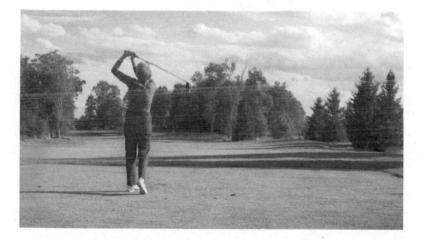

COMMENT: Marcy's trials and tribulations remind us once again that typically many different factors conspire to effect cognitive decline, and the set of factors is different for each person. Marcy was low in numerous nutrients and hormones, so she had features of type 2 Alzheimer's (atrophic), and she addressed this problem successfully. However, with additional tests, it turned out that she also had exposure to multiple toxins (type 3 Alzheimer's), from metals like mercury to organic toxins to biotoxins.

It is worth commenting on Marcy's point that she may have been exposed to toxins while playing golf. Several different physicians have commented on something that might be called "golf course syndrome"—it is relatively common for people who are living on golf courses or spending a great deal of time on golf courses to complain of cognitive decline. This may turn out to be unrelated to the golf courses themselves, and in fact golf is a wonderful exercise and exercise is an important preventive measure for cognitive decline. However, just to be safe, if you spend large amounts of time on or near a golf course, please simply have your toxin levels checked, including for toxic pesticides.

In addition to the toxins discovered, it turned out that Marcy also had exposure to *Borrelia* (the Lyme disease organism) and *Ehrlichia*, both of which are injected during tick bites. These organisms can live in our bodies for many years, and often go undiagnosed. It is the ongoing "cold war" with these long-term pathogens like *Herpes*, *Borrelia*, *Ehrlichia*, and *Babesia* that leads to the protective response of Alzheimer's-associated amyloid, since the amyloid kills microorganisms.

Despite her infections, Marcy's most recent MRI showed an increase in volume of her hippocampus, which fits very well with her cognitive improvement. In addition, her follow-up PET scan showed improvement, and was no longer felt to be compatible with Alzheimer's disease.

Now that Marcy has reversed her cognitive decline, the key is to continue to optimize, in order to enhance the improvement she has enjoyed already. Is there any contributor that has been missed? Can she achieve an optimal level of ketones? Is she optimally insulin sensitive? Is her gut microbiome what it should be? And so on. As you'll see from Sally's story next, continuing to tweak your program is often very helpful.

CHAPTER 5

Sally's Story:
A Failed Trial

You may have to fight a battle more than once to win it.

—MARGARET THATCHER

As a gerontological nursing professor, I taught that Alzheimer's disease cannot be prevented or reversed. My personal experience is proving otherwise. For the past five years, I've been reversing my symptoms of early Alzheimer's. It continues to be a daily struggle, but it's working!

Five years ago, I often could not remember the day of the week. Even worse, I sometimes forgot to pick up my granddaughters to take them to school and often mixed up their names. On a cognitive test, I scored "mildly cognitively impaired," which means that I was well on the way to having Alzheimer's disease. Asked to draw a clock face, I had trouble remembering whether the hour hand was the short one or the long one. A PET brain scan revealed that I had beta-amyloid plaques associated with Alzheimer's.

I enrolled in a clinical trial to remove the amyloid, but with each injection of the drug, my memory worsened instead of improving. Therefore, after eight treatments, I decided to drop out of the trial.

My husband heard about Dr. Bredesen's research on a public talk show. I contacted Dr. Bredesen to ask if I could be part of his research study. His answer was no, since I did not live near the study's sites in California. However, he offered to share information on his Reversal of Cognitive Decline (ReCODE) program with my doctor and me. My first step was to complete a cognoscopy—a panel of thirty-six blood and genetic tests to assess specific risk factors for Alzheimer's. I was horrified to find out that I was positive on almost all thirty-six indicators. In fact, I was pretty unusual, since I had risk factors for five of the six types of Alzheimer's that Dr. Bredesen had identified, especially the toxic type. Furthermore, I tested positive for ApoE4—I had one copy of that so-called Alzheimer's risk gene.

The steps that I needed to take seemed overwhelming at first, so I decided to focus on making one change at a time. Now, five years later, I have implemented all of the ReCODE program and my brain continues to improve:

- My brain remembers to keep my cell phone close by.
- My brain reminds me to bring my driver's license and my credit cards when I leave home.
- My brain can problem-solve how to cook a meal for my children and their families.
- My brain enjoys brain-training games.
- My brain remembers what day it is.
- Most important of all, I remember to pick up my granddaughters and take them to school!

My current "thinking" brain is a result of fully and consistently implementing the ReCODE program for the last five years. About half of the thirty-six indicators returned to the normal range during my second year of ReCODE, and I continue to improve with each subsequent cognoscopy. Now I consistently get a perfect (or near-perfect) score of 30/30 on the Montreal Cognitive Assessment Test (MoCA), after starting at only 24.5. I am delighted that my cognitive score on the much more rigorous computerized neurocognitive assessment CNS Vital Signs was above average on 7 out of the 10 indicators after four years of following the ReCODE program.

I've gone from fear, dread, and sadness to hope and joy. I can realistically dream that even many years from now, I will still be able to call all of my six grandchildren by their correct names. I used to take my brain for granted, but no more.

My inflammatory blood values are now in the normal range, indicating I have eliminated type 1 (inflammatory) as an underlying cause of Alzheimer's. Similarly, I have eliminated type 1.5 (glycotoxic) as an underlying cause of Alzheimer's. And my current lab values indicate that I have made significant progress in improving both type 2 (atrophic) and type 3 (toxic) as risk factors for Alzheimer's. As for type 5 (traumatic Alzheimer's), the supplements and lifestyle changes I have made over the last five years have addressed my key neurochemistry associated with synapse formation.

Initially, on many days, I found it hard to follow the ReCODE program due to the required time and expense (of some of the supplements), as well as the need to change lifestyle habits. I often wished that my remaining lab values would become normal faster. I often felt like I was improving at the speed of a tortoise. When I needed encouragement, I would remind myself that the tortoise won the proverbial race.

From year one to now, in year five of the ReCODE program, I tell myself it's a "no-brainer": I remind myself that a brain is a terrible thing to lose—especially when it's yours! I am going to keep on the program so that I can keep my brain. I sometimes wish that Dr. Bredesen's ReCODE program had been available when I was in my 40s, but today, at age 74, I am grateful for my chance to maintain my functioning brain.

RESPONSES TO ALZHEIMER'S

The discussion that follows is organized into four stages:

1. Early stage: Fear, lack of awareness, and denial
2. Middle stage: Awareness and reversal of early symptoms
3. Current stage: Reversal process and optimization
4. Future stage: Dream and anticipation

My transitions from one stage to the next have seldom been linear. Mostly, my progress has been up and down, with improvements and regressions at each stage. And in practice, all of the stages overlap with each other.

Early-Stage Responses to Alzheimer's

Early stage: fear. Since my early 40s, I have been afraid of Alzheimer's. My mother's two sisters were surrogate mothers to me when my own biological mother was unable to care for me. My heart broke as I watched my two aunts develop Alzheimer's, deteriorate gradually, and eventually die from the disease. Alzheimer's was also painfully familiar on my father's side, with both an aunt and an uncle dying from Alzheimer's.

I had specialized in gerontology early in my career as a registered nurse and a professor of nursing. I had cared for Alzheimer's patients in nursing homes and in-home settings, and observed firsthand how the needs of persons with Alzheimer's usually exceed the time and abilities of both loved ones and health professionals. I saw directly that there are no easy answers for Alzheimer's patients or their families.

Early stage: lack of awareness. My own stage of being personally "unaware" of my Alzheimer's began over twenty years ago, when I developed severe depression. At the time, I attributed it to menopause and an interstate move to a new, stressful, and challenging position at a new university. I attributed my depression to how much I missed seeing my family regularly. My doctor prescribed an antidepressant, which did at least relieve my symptoms. What I could not have known in 2000 was that depression is a common early symptom of type 3 Alzheimer's. During the next twenty plus years, I experienced intermittent acute episodes of depression, often following a change of location or a physical injury. I was aware that I had trouble thinking clearly during this time, but I attributed my cognitive changes to my depression and "normal" aging. Back when I had taught gerontology to nursing students, I had told them the prevailing theory that one cause of memory loss was depression (pseudodementia), and that once the depression was treated, the memory loss would be eliminated.

Only after reading Dr. Bredesen's 2016 publication about type 3

Alzheimer's and inhalational toxins did I realize that the home I had lived in for five years had almost certainly contributed to my Alzheimer's and depression. My home had an untreated mold-infested basement. It was also much too close to a busy interstate highway, and the fumes were so strong that my husband's eyes and my own would burn in the late afternoons and evenings.

When I had my first cognoscopy, I learned that my genes put me in the 25 percent of the population that finds it nearly impossible to fight off inhalational toxins such as mold, or chemical and microparticulate pollution. I realized that I was positive on twelve of Dr. Bredesen's fifteen characteristics for type 3 Alzheimer's. Today, after treatment for the underlying cause—inhalational toxins—I am no longer depressed, and many of my abnormal blood values that indicate toxicity have returned to normal. Nevertheless, type 3 Alzheimer's is very difficult to treat, and several of my toxicity exposure blood values continue to be abnormal. I have accepted that I will probably always be hypersensitive to mold exposure and will need to avoid high-risk environments even though they do not cause problems for most others. Today, I am glad that others like me, those who are genetically unable to fight off toxins, have effective treatments available, and can detect their vulnerability earlier and more readily than I could.

Early stage: denial. Approximately twelve years ago, my hands started moving in random, jerky, uncontrollable ways when I was sitting still. I had observed the same random hand movement in Alzheimer's patients in a nursing home care unit where I worked, and also in my own aunt when she got Alzheimer's. My conscious mind said *Alzheimer's*, but at some level, I refused to recognize the possibility, stayed in denial, and just refused to think about it. My realization that I was in denial of my Alzheimer's was heightened when I fell asleep in a car, and the driver, my coworker, said, "You must have played the piano." At the time, I remember thinking to myself, *Oh no! This means Alzheimer's. I don't want to have Alzheimer's!*

Around the same time, I started using the wrong word frequently, often causing confusion for my listeners. I told them that I had developed aphasia associated with aging. I truly believed this myself. This issue continues, but only when I am tired or am trying to carry on a conversation while I complete a task requiring several steps. For example, once, when I was preparing dinner for my son and his family I said, "For safety, I have given up using my cell phone while talking" (instead of *driving*). I now recognize the use of incorrect words for what it really is: an indicator of Alzheimer's risk, and of the need to continue ReCODE to retain my cognition.

I am so grateful that my healthy lifestyle may have postponed the onset of my Alzheimer's for long enough for Dr. Bredesen's ReCODE treatment to become available. For the last forty years, I have followed a cancer-prevention diet, including lots of fruits and vegetables, plenty of greens, minimal animal fat, and daily green tea. I took daily supplements from a reputable distributor aimed at slowing aging and preventing Alzheimer's.

I also exercised regularly—anywhere from 30 to 60 minutes a day, at least five days per week. During my 50s and 60s, I backpacked 1,741 miles on the Appalachian Trail.

My own symptoms first appeared earlier in life than they did for my relatives in the previous generation. This earlier age onset is typical of type 3 Alzheimer's. I am convinced that my healthy diet and physical exercise helped delay the onset of my Alzheimer's. That delay bought me precious time—time for Dr. Bredesen to develop ReCODE through his laboratory research, and later, time for me to learn about and implement ReCODE's lifesaving changes.

Middle-Stage Responses to Alzheimer's

Middle stage: awareness. Five years ago, twice within a month I forgot that I was scheduled to pick up my grandchildren and take them to school. I could no longer attribute my memory losses to normal aging changes. My initial score of 24.5/30 on the Montreal Cognitive Assessment Test documented that I had mild cognitive impairment. This was also the time when a PET scan revealed beta-amyloid plaques in my brain, and I was told that I was developing Alzheimer's disease.

I was at a loss as to what to do, since there was no treatment for Alzheimer's disease at the time. Back then, beta-amyloid plaques were believed to predict probable Alzheimer's within ten to fifteen years. I did not want to gradually die from Alzheimer's the way my loved ones had.

I told myself I would not keep living if I developed Alzheimer's disease, but taking my life was not a choice for me, either. I might have considered suicide, but I had seen what it had cost my extended family and friends in two separate cases. I would not have been willing to put my family through the pain those two families had experienced. My family had assured me that they would take care of me if I ever did develop Alzheimer's. While I treasured their reassurance, I still felt hopeless.

Meanwhile, my cognitive impairment led to difficulties with many everyday tasks, including computer work, shopping, and cooking. I had trouble remembering names and was embarrassed several times when I stopped in the middle of a sentence, unable to recall my topic. I had trouble making a gingerbread man with my granddaughter, even though I had done it several times before with two older granddaughters. My self-awareness of these cognitive problems was painful.

Middle stage: reversal. As a researcher, I actively sought studies for treatment and/or prevention of cognitive decline. I enrolled in a nationwide study of a promising Alzheimer's drug six years ago, one that was targeted to remove the amyloid plaques. However, after each monthly injection, rather than improving, I experienced increased confusion and anxiety for three to five days. During eight months of treatment, I became aware that my cognition was becoming worse instead of staying the same or improving. I was losing the battle.

Then five years ago, I contacted Dr. Bredesen after my husband heard him on a radio talk show. I started implementing his ReCODE program. At first, I was overwhelmed by all the different elements of the program. I decided to implement ReCODE one step at a time, taking time to observe my reaction after each step. I started to make the following changes:

Sleep. I gradually increased my sleep from about six hours per night to an average of seven or eight hours. Sleep continues to be enhanced when I (1) lower the bedroom lights before bed; (2) avoid electronic media two hours before bedtime; (3) meditate during the day; (4) stretch my muscles during the day; and (5) avoid political or other difficult discussions two hours before bedtime. Several supplements, including melatonin, also improve my sleep quality and duration.

Diet. I had avoided eating organic foods due to their cost. When I began to follow the ReCODE program and ate vegetables and fruit in the Environmental Working Group's Dirty Dozen category, I bought organic only. It took me a full year to implement this completely, because cost and availability meant that I had to reduce consumption of many of my favorite foods—especially sweet peppers, a mainstay snack for me. I added lemon juice to water and drank it first thing in the morning. I now carry raw nuts—all kinds—with me as a quick and easy snack when I am not at home. Organic seaweed is another snack option that is rich in nutrients. I usually keep an extra package in the car.

More recently, after reading Dr. Bredesen's 2020 book, *The End of Alzheimer's Program*, I am paying more attention to ensure intake of foods that are prebiotic, probiotic, or contain resistant starches. I now eat food sources from two out of these three categories daily.

Meditation and exercise. These led to cognitive improvement that came swiftly and was easy to observe. That was not the case for dietary changes—those improvements took over six months before I was able to observe them. But over time, the improvements were unmistakable, and my ability to think clearly has significantly improved. I believe that following the ReCODE program for dietary intake is an essential part of the program.

Ketogenesis. I had a lot of frustration implementing a ketogenic diet. After six months of trying and failing, I realized my failure was due to two supplements I was taking—one for intestinal permeability, the other for my type 3 Alzheimer's. Both supplements had sugar in them. Once I readjusted with other supplements, I became ketogenic. I now achieve mild ketogenesis on most days. The days I do not, I observe decreased cognition, usually within twenty-four hours. Most days, my brain wins out over my stomach—unless I'm tired, when the stomach wins the battle. I then pay the negative consequences of a decreased ability to think. There were added benefits of the ketogenic diet that I had not expected. I lost ten pounds without trying. Also, I am no longer hungry all the time, which I thoroughly enjoy.

Current-Stage Responses to Alzheimer's

Today, my negative feelings about Alzheimer's have diminished and been replaced with many positive feelings that include appreciation, gratitude, hope, and a desire to help others. My earlier poor score on the MoCA cognitive test has improved to a perfect 30/30. I have a strong appreciation for Dr. Bredesen and his ReCODE Protocol, and gratitude for helpful family members, friends, and physicians. I have hope in my future—hope that I can delay or prevent Alzheimer's. My daily life is full of joy. With recovery, I can think more clearly and act on my lifetime desire to help others. Formerly, with impaired thinking, I became self-focused, as even minor tasks were hard to accomplish. Normal activities like cooking took all my energy and time, leading to a sense of incompleteness and frustration.

Current stage: reversal. Dr. Bredesen is correct when he writes that type 3 (toxic) Alzheimer's is harder to treat than type 1 (inflammatory) or type 2 (atrophic). My treatment for type 3 Alzheimer's was difficult due to my rare, highly susceptible HLA haplotype (immune-system genetics). I found it quite difficult to fight off inhalational toxins when I was exposed to them. Any time that I was exposed to indoor environments that had not had mold remediation, I reacted with symptoms of chronic inflammatory response syndrome (CIRS). My CIRS symptoms include brain fog, joint pain, vertigo, breathing difficulties, depression, and even anxiety.

Continued reversal and prevention of these symptoms required caution and prudence, along with a lot of discipline. To avoid these symptoms, I lived in a kind of self-imposed homebound status. I avoided visits to most other indoor environments. I enjoyed spending a lot of time outdoors, in the fresh air.

During years two and three of ReCODE, while I was following the Shoemaker Protocol for the mold toxins of type 3 Alzheimer's, I missed many of the social activities that I have always enjoyed, including attending church, group Pilates sessions, eating in restaurants, and—saddest of all—visiting friends and relatives in their homes. I often was frustrated or felt overwhelmed by the complexity of type 3 Alzheimer's treatment. But still, I knew beyond a shadow of doubt that the benefits for my functioning brain greatly outweighed the costs. I can greet people by name, I can carry on conversations, and I remember what I need to do to get ready for activities such as swimming, boating, or walking. Before ReCODE, I had difficulty making basic decisions, such as what to wear or what to take with me.

Year four of ReCODE, to increase my ability to go into other indoor environments without negative physical and mental reactions, I started the Dynamic Neural Retraining System (DNRS). DNRS is a natural drug-free neuroplasticity-based program discussed in Dr. Bredesen's 2020 book. I was making significant progress and had increased my indoor environmental exposures to several locations, including my granddaughters' homes, church, Pilates studio, and friends' homes. Then the COVID-19 pandemic started, and my interval training to other indoor environments stopped for the duration of the pandemic. I look forward to continued increased exposure to other indoor environments once the pandemic is over.

As I progress through year five of ReCODE, I continue my daily hour practice of a DNRS mental exercise. The mental exercises consist of self-messages with positive visualizations designed to remind my limbic system to remain calm and not react with the negative symptoms. These include visualizing a positive past experience in great detail. Then I apply the positive feelings and thoughts from my past experience to an imagined future experience, visualizing my future experience as vividly as possible. These positive memories—both past and future—flood my brain and body with positive hormones of dopamine, oxytocin, serotonin, and endorphins. These hormones have been shown to promote neuroplasticity, healing, and growth in brain cells. But even more important, these visualizations enable me to experience hope and support my dream of an Alzheimer's-free future. This is in contrast to the negative hormones of cortisol, adrenaline, and norepinephrine that have a negative impact on my brain cells when and if I let my brain focus on fear of Alzheimer's and/or negative thoughts.

Some other adjustments that I have had to make to stay on my course of reversal:

Cost. My husband and I struggle with the expenses associated with treating type 3 Alzheimer's. We are making difficult decisions about what we can and cannot afford. However, we never forget that our current costs are far less than the high cost for Alzheimer's care in a nursing home.

Meditation. Meditation in the form of prayer, for thirty minutes each morning, was the first lifestyle behavior I changed my first year of ReCODE. One month later, I was experiencing more peace and joy, as well as better cognition.

Today, in year five of ReCODE, I continue to value my twice-a-day meditation time, which I spend alone talking and listening to God, reading the Bible, or listening to religious music. My husband also reads a daily devotion to me, which we both thoroughly enjoy. I am surprised, therefore, that this four-year habit of daily meditation is hard to maintain. When I have a full day's activity, I often think, *I don't have time for thirty minutes now.* But after several days of only short meditations, I find myself dragging emotionally; when I refocus and take time for meditating, I once again become refreshed and revived. I suppose that we all find ourselves at times taking actions that are not in our best interest in the long run, but feel good in the short run. I have come to realize that successful adherence to ReCODE is a long-term decision, one that involves many short-term decisions and actions.

When Dr. Bredesen's 2020 book was published, I read his recommendations for mindfulness, the practice of being fully present in each moment. Now I am learning to have increased focus on today, an acceptance of things as they are, and being in an observer's frame of mind. I experience joy as a result of these personal changes. I see parallels between mindfulness and one of my favorite Bible verses, from Matthew 6:34: "Therefore, do not worry about tomorrow, for tomorrow will worry about itself. Each day has enough trouble of its own."

Brain training. Five years ago, I almost caused two car accidents that would have been my fault. Only the other drivers' actions prevented the accidents. I began to practice the BrainHQ exercises (especially Double Decision, which has been shown to improve safe driving). My driving skills have clearly improved, and I now play Brain HQ for at least thirty minutes per day, five or six times per week. As is true with meditation, it is easy for me to find other things I need to do before I take time to do brain training. I continue to be amazed at how easy it is for me not to do what I need to do, even though conceptually, I would do whatever it takes to keep my well-functioning brain. Using a checklist to track my daily BrainHQ sessions has helped me remain consistent.

Exercise. Dr. Bredesen recommends exercise of at least thirty minutes per day, at least five days a week. Since I was already doing this, I increased the time and intensity of my exercise my first year of ReCODE. I immediately saw further improvements in cognition.

Today, in year five with ReCODE, I have knee challenges with walking on hard pavement, but I continue to be able to walk in the woods. I also enjoy swimming, kayaking, and practicing Pilates and yoga. I have had seven different orthopedic injuries and three surgeries. I am an orthopedic example of what a person can do if one keeps moving, despite major injuries. I continue to notice that my cognition is better on the days when I get more exercise.

Feelings. My overall feeling about Alzheimer's now is hope—hope that my cognition continues to improve and hope that, when I do die someday, it shall be of something other than Alzheimer's. I do not fear death; in fact, as a Christian, I look forward to time with God. But I am choosing to follow the ReCODE program so that I avoid the slow death that comes with Alzheimer's. Today, when I wake up in the morning, I experience joy rather than depression and anxiety. I treasure my time with my husband, family, and friends. I say, "Thank you!" every time I can remember someone's name. Many of my negative feelings about Alzheimer's have disappeared. I am living proof that slow, confused thinking can be reversed.

Current stage: optimization. To carry out Dr. Bredesen's ReCODE program fully and effectively, I use several techniques, including reminders and research on the web. Post-it Notes on my bathroom mirror or kitchen counter, alarms on my phone, and checkoffs on my calendar help make new practices become regular habits (and there is a new app). Research on the web helps me understand the consequences of what I am doing and gives me knowledge on what to observe.

Electronic notes about my symptoms and treatment for type 3 Alzheimer's have been critical for maintaining and improving my treatment. Based on Dr. Bredesen's recommendations, I followed Dr. Ritchie Shoemaker's twelve-step protocol to remove the bio-toxins from my body and help reduce my inhalational sensitivity symptoms. I began Dr. Shoemaker's protocol, including intake of cholestyramine, four years ago. I finished the final step, vasoactive intestinal peptide (VIP), during year three of my ReCODE program. I believe the two years and four months that I took to complete the Shoemaker Protocol took several times longer than what is typical for most patients, though I do not have reliable data to make the comparison. The VIP treatment was quite expensive and labor-intensive, and health insurance does not cover this treatment. The good news is that I no longer have symptoms of chronic inflammatory response syndrome (CIRS), unless I have new toxic exposures. For the last year and a half, I have avoided CIRS symptoms: depression, anxiety, achy joints, brain fog, dizziness, and tight chest congestion.

I have increased my intake of green leafy vegetables by making multiple green smoothies at one time. In addition to organic spinach and kale, I include healthy vegetables from the refrigerator plus cinnamon, vanilla, small amounts of blueberries, and rice and pea protein powder. I may include herbs such as cilantro and mint. I freeze each smoothie in a single-size container with a lid. Then I can pull out a green smoothie each day and have a concentrated quantity of green leafy vegetable plus other healthy nutrients.

Some other ways that I have optimized:

Supplements. Initially, the multiple supplements that are part of Dr. Bredesen's ReCODE program were overwhelming to me. I decided to start each supplement one day at a time. For about two weeks, I studied the possible side effects. I found that I was able to take all the supplements except two. Curcumin 1 gram, taken twice a day, led to bruising that went away when I decreased the dosage and frequency to once a day. Liposomal glutathione (for type 3 Alzheimer's) gave me nausea. Initially, I reduced the dosage of glutathione. After one year, I successfully increased the dosage and took it with powdered ginger in a drink.

The first four years of the ReCODE program, I individually ordered each supplement from reputable distributors. This was very confusing, as I did not know which distributor was the most reliable for which supplements. Year four, I found and used ConsumerLab.com to evaluate each supplement and distributor.

Preparing my daily supplements had been quite time consuming. Ordering the supplements from LifeSeasons (lifeseasons .com) has recently become available, and I look forward to obtaining many of my supplements—premixed, and in all the right dosages—through them. I am glad that future ReCODE participants will have this convenient and reliable source for obtaining their supplements.

The positive effects from my supplements were gradual and cumulative. When in preparation for surgery I had to stop all supplements for two weeks, though, I did not yet know that

Dr. Bredesen recommends stopping them gradually, and I stopped taking them all at once. I then experienced a clear decrease in cognition. Once I resumed my supplements following surgery, it took almost a year for me to reach my previous state of cognition. Hence, I continue to be a strong believer in the benefits of the supplements.

Anesthesia. Another contributor to my decreased cognition following surgery was undergoing general anesthesia. I learned from Dr. Bredesen's book that anesthesia can have a negative impact on cognition for persons like me with previous mild cognitive impairment. Therefore, a year ago, when I had surgery on my knee, I requested and received spinal anesthesia instead of general anesthesia and did not experience any cognitive loss at all following surgery.

Coping. I use several strategies daily to cope with the challenges I face. These include meditation with a focus on prayer, social support, humor, and exercise. It's easy to let negative thoughts slip into consciousness. When they do, I replace them with positive thoughts. I've also found that humor is very effective in coping with these stresses. I tell jokes and ask others to tell me their favorites. Deliberately choosing an optimistic attitude helps. I used to feel discouraged, but now my inner dialogue is that my cup is half full, instead of half empty. When I am inadvertently exposed to inhalational toxins, I focus on what is working, instead of thinking about what does not.

But my strongest source of support is my deep faith in God and Jesus, and experiencing their unconditional love and caring for me. In fact, my experiences while reversing early symptoms of Alzheimer's have strengthened that faith and trust. A favorite Bible verse is Jeremiah 29:11: "'For I know the plans I have for you,' declares the Lord, 'plans to prosper you and not to harm you, plans to give you hope and a future.'"

Future-Stage Responses to Alzheimer's

Future stage: dream. I realize that it's possible I may only delay Alzheimer's substantially, without avoiding it completely in my lifetime. But for me, my current strategy of dreaming of a positive future makes the best sense.

On the rare occasions when I allow myself to think of what my brain could be like in fifteen years, I feel a deep dread and fear of Alzheimer's. Unfortunately, the early part of my career, as a gerontological nurse, only deepens that fear. When these negative thoughts occur, I remind myself that I choose to continue to live a healthy life and follow the ReCODE program. And that this increases the chances that when I do die, it will be from something other than Alzheimer's. I then deliberately switch my brain to a different, more positive thought.

My dream is that by continuing the ReCODE program, I will be able to avoid Alzheimer's—no matter what age I am or how old I live to be. This new dream is still fragile, but I am convinced that the more I live this dream, practice this dream, and believe this dream, the more likely it is to become true. I can realistically dream of a future without Alzheimer's. Where my thoughts go, my brain, mind, and body will follow. I am enjoying learning about the promises of neuroplasticity. I love having a healthy brain that thinks clearly and remembers things. And I commit to faithfully follow the ReCODE program. A healthy working brain is worth it!

Future stage: anticipation. The title for part one, "It Tolls for

Thee No More," holds a special meaning for me. In 1953, during the Korean War, when I was 5 years old, my father's plane crashed on takeoff from an aircraft carrier. Unfortunately, his body was never recovered. John Donne's poem "For Whom the Bell Tolls" was a part of his memorial service. As my father's death diminished us all, I pray that my defeat of Alzheimer's can in contrast enhance the life of others and give them hope.

In year five of my ReCODE program, I can anticipate and visualize the next fifteen years. And like an 86-year-old friend who recently led a New Year's Eve COVID Zoom party, I am active, have a clear, thinking mind, and hopefully, am a joy to be around. I smile when I anticipate future old age and "time marching on." For I now anticipate a future—a future without Alzheimer's. In my mind's eye, I see both my earthly father and my spiritual father smiling from heaven. And I am smiling right back! Thanks to the ReCODE program, Alzheimer's tolls for me no more!

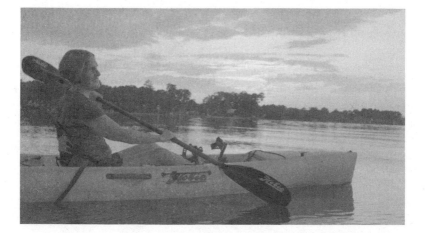

COMMENT: Over the past few years, I have come to realize that the protocol my colleagues and I developed for cognitive decline is actually more like surgery than medicine, and Sally's story illustrates that point. In other words, rather than attacking the disease process with a prescription, one must identify the various contributors and then follow a targeted, stepwise program—much more like a surgical procedure than the medicine of the twentieth century. However, as Sally's results, and those of so many others show, this precision medicine programmatic approach produces results that have never been achieved with simple prescriptive medicine.

Sally's clinical course illustrates another potentially important point: although her PET scan showed the amyloid and thus supported a diagnosis of Alzheimer's disease, when she was treated with a drug that targets and removes amyloid, she clearly worsened with each injection, rather than improving or even remaining stable. We have observed this phenomenon with a number of patients now, with clear worsening linked temporally to anti-amyloid injections. Since beta-amyloid has an antimicrobial effect, this is understandable, and once again suggests that it may make most sense to remove the pathogens first, prior to administering the anti-amyloid therapy.

CHAPTER 6

Frank's Story:
Señor Moments

The opportunity to secure ourselves against defeat lies in our own hands,
but the opportunity of defeating the enemy
is provided by the enemy himself.

—SUN TZU

ast February I was at a doctor's office with my wife. We were trying to get some billing information translated into English for insurance purposes. The secretary asked me if I could remember the dates of the last two visits. I thought about it for a second and without hesitation said, "December twenty-sixth and January fifteenth."

No big deal, right? For a guy who was diagnosed with early-onset Alzheimer's nine years ago, it was huge. It was one more incident proving that the Bredesen Protocol is indeed reversing the symptoms of my disease.

At the time I was diagnosed it was a big deal for me if I could remember to zip up my pants and buckle my belt before leaving the house. That would be after twenty minutes of trying to find my keys and my phone. I found my phone in the refrigerator one morning.

Six years ago, we moved to Mexico, convinced that I would soon need more care than my wife could provide or we could afford.

I think my wife suspected I had dementia long before I was willing to admit it to myself. She was seeing the destruction I was wreaking on my once-successful business and our personal finances. Eventually the evidence became so overwhelming that I was convinced I must have Alzheimer's. Still I sought no medical help.

I had put it off for a couple of reasons. It was 2011. Most of the world had yet to hear of Dr. Bredesen. It was a few years before his first study was presented to the world. At that point almost everyone agreed Alzheimer's was fatal and incurable. I didn't even know how to spell the word, but I knew that I was going to die from it.

That thinking kept me from seeking any help for a very long time. My strategy had been to try and hide the multiple mistakes I was making on a daily basis and hope no one would notice.

There was another thing going on. I could not remember much of what was occurring. I would borrow money from myself to complete company projects, thinking I would repay the loan at the project's completion. By the time it was done I would forget that I had borrowed money to complete it. It created an illusion of the company being okay.

I had been seeing a doctor for depression, a psychiatrist. When I finally told him I thought I had Alzheimer's, he said I was too young. I didn't know back then that there were many varieties of dementia and many stages of Alzheimer's. The doctor believed my problem was that I was still severely depressed and adjusted my medication. It was a good idea. The depression lifted a great deal, but my memory continued to decline.

After some standard cognitive tests, he agreed that I might have mild cognitive impairment. I must have been driving him crazy. I kept saying, "There is nothing mild about what is happening to my life."

He may have been right. I have often wondered why I did not immediately google memory loss and find out a few things. I guess I just didn't believe there was anything good to be found.

Eventually, in 2012, I was diagnosed with early-onset Alzheimer's. I had been taking notes of the bizarre things I was doing every day. I was going to write a book called *Descent into Dementia,* chronicling the whole thing for as long as I could.

When we moved to Mexico, I was convinced it was only a matter of time before I would be such a drain on my wife I would have to execute the "final solution," which I had acquired the means to do several months before.

We had been in Mexico less than a year when I had the great good fortune to overhear a conversation about Dr. Bredesen. He had just released the results of his study with the first ten subjects. I googled the report and was stunned to find that some of the case studies were people experiencing exactly what I had been going through. I knew that somehow I needed to meet the man. I also started trying to do the same things the people in the case studies had done.

After several months and many emails, I got him on the phone. His secretary told me I would be lucky to get five minutes of his time. It was a Friday afternoon. We spoke for twenty-five minutes. I told him my experience and the fact that I had been writing a book about what was happening to me. I was asking for a face-to-face interview. I also told him I was seeing some improvement after trying his protocol.

He did most of the talking, asking me questions. He seemed more interested in my case than any of my own doctors. He invited me to his lab in Marin County, where he was putting on a presentation of his protocol. He said there would be someone there that I should meet.

I was still very ill, and the idea of traveling alone to California was frightening. It ended up being the best thing I ever did. After his presentation, we spoke for about half an hour, during which he explained the protocol in simple terms that I could understand, and he answered all of my questions. It was the beginning of regaining my life. I met a woman who'd had the exact same symptoms as I had and had completely recovered. She was sharp as a tack. She made me a believer. I left California committed to giving the protocol everything I had. And I took with me something I had left behind years ago: *hope.*

Eventually I started feeling more and more like myself. I had a relapse in my second year. Away from home doing some business at the border, I binged on junk food the whole time. Three pounds of licorice, McDonald's, a huge jar of peanut butter, about six or seven large cinnamon rolls, and several milk shakes. I gained five pounds in three days.

Okay, I gained the weight. Bad enough by itself. Unfortunately it led me back to eating the junk food I had lived on for years. Without even knowing it, I'd stopped taking my supplements and exercising. It didn't take long. I ended up unable to hold a thought and once again terrified.

I made a phone call to someone who knew much more about the protocol than I did. He told me it wasn't uncommon for people to fall off the wagon. More important, he told me most of them were able to regain their cognition.

It was harder the second time. It seemed to take longer. But eventually I was once again myself. Have I been cured? I look at it the way alcoholics look at sobriety. As long as they don't drink, their lives are like those of other men or women. If they go back to the booze, they go back to misery. That is how I feel about Alzheimer's. As long as I continue to follow the protocol, I have a normal life. If I don't, the nightmare will begin all over.

If you are wondering if you can do it, I am here to tell you that you can. Can your loved one do it? With your help, there is a good chance she can. First, get the testing done so you know what you need to address. Then start where you are able. For me, the change of diet was the hardest. I never knew how much I loved sugar and bread. I rarely ate salads or fish, even when living in the Caribbean. I have been learning more about the protocol and adding things to my daily plan for as long as I have been doing it. It would have been impossible to do so without my wife. In the beginning I had to be reminded every day to take my supplements.

I have been thinking clearly for the majority of the last four plus years. I realize now that my problems in cognition started much earlier than I originally thought. In my mid-50s I was having occasional incidents that I simply chose to ignore or blamed on stress.

Do not do what I did. Do not delay seeking help. The sooner you address your problems or start living a healthier life even if you do not yet experience problems, the better a life you will have. The protocol prevents the disease. You do not need to go where I went.

Oh, I finished the book. *Descent into Dementia* ended up being *Defeating Dementia,* and with Dr. Bredesen's endorsement, I like to believe it has helped spread the message to many lands. I remain forever grateful.

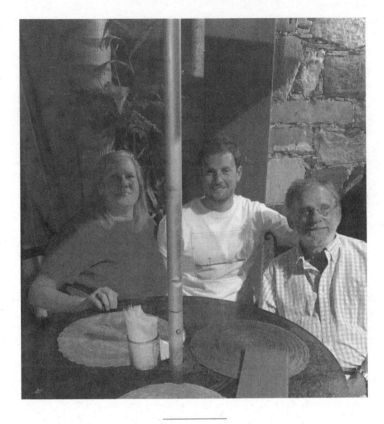

COMMENT: Frank's story illustrates the most important point of all, one that has been echoed by many other patients: improvement is sustained when you are targeting the actual insults causing the cognitive decline rather than trying to circumvent the causes by using a single drug alone. How long can we sustain these improvements? We know the answer is at least nine years (since the first patients began the protocol nine years ago), but since the underlying neurochemistry has been corrected, there is every reason to believe that these improvements will continue for decades to come. Can we create a global program to allow everyone to stay sharp until 90 or 100, avoiding dementia? That is the goal.

CHAPTER 7

Julie's Story:
Good Luck with That

The amount of good luck coming your way
depends on your willingness to act.

—BARBARA SHER

O n the cusp of my 50th birthday, instead of planning a celebration, I came face-to-face with my own mortality. For several years, I'd been experiencing odd, debilitating, seemingly unrelated medical symptoms. My physicians were at a loss to explain them. I thought participating in genetic testing might yield some helpful clues. I sent out to 23andMe, a direct-to-consumer genetic testing service, for a kit. Once it arrived, I spit in a test tube, mailed off the sample, and waited. Several weeks later, my results arrived by email. I logged onto the site and skimmed through my results. To my untrained eye, absolutely nothing was remarkable; phew.

Then at the very end, one set of results required me to check off a series of boxes and view a video. It was for a gene associated with Alzheimer's disease. I knew little about Alzheimer's and (at that point) wasn't aware of any family history. I leaped ahead, checked off all the boxes, pretended I'd watched the video, and opened up my results. They weren't good. In fact, they were very bad. I learned I was among a tiny segment of the population (less than 2 percent—nearly 7 million Americans) that carries two copies of the epsilon 4 version of the APOE gene. I'd never even heard of this gene before, but I quickly engaged in a crash course to learn all that I could.

Some of the statistics for ApoE4 homozygotes (people who carry two copies of ApoE4) were quite dire, suggesting that I had a greater than 90 percent chance of developing Alzheimer's disease in my lifetime. Even worse, researchers sometimes describe ApoE4 as the "frailty" gene. Carriers are predisposed not only to Alzheimer's and other dementias but also to heart disease, and they tend to have shortened lifespans. In my research, I stumbled upon an anecdote about James Watson, the co-discoverer of the structure of DNA. He had his own genome sequenced but decided to opt out of learning about *one* gene: APOE. Knowledge that he might carry one copy of ApoE4, much less two, was more than he could bear. The consensus at that time was that nothing could be done to mitigate risk. The full implication of everything I was learning was beginning to sink in.

This was over eight years ago. I turned to the Alzheimer's Association for more information. Their website stated that Alzheimer's disease was incurable, untreatable, and progressive. On average, patients died within ten years of symptom onset. Most frightening to me was their claim that Alzheimer's couldn't be prevented. Around this same time, my cousin was diagnosed with Alzheimer's based upon symptoms and his cerebral spinal fluid results. I thought of the disease as something that affected only older people, but my cousin was several months *younger* than I was. His experience brought this threat, that I initially thought might be my future, into my present reality. I was officially paralyzed with terror.

I was having some cognitive issues at the time, but I'd been attributing them to stress, perimenopause, my busy lifestyle—anything but Alzheimer's. Simply for reassurance, I decided to do some cognitive testing through an online brain-training website. I'd always learned easily and was an excellent student. I was stunned to find I had scored in the mid-30th percentile for my age group.

I repeated the testing several times, only to get the same result. I turned to my husband, my rock, for reassurance that I was blowing this out of proportion. I told him about my high genetic risk for Alzheimer's disease and my poor score on cognitive testing. Instead of comforting me, he said, "*Well, that explains a lot!*" My initial response was to be angry with him. How could he not reassure me? But he was worried, too. Bruce is an international airline pilot and he's often away from home for up to a week at a time. He was becoming concerned about how much further I had declined each time he returned from a trip.

I was forced to take a hard look at myself and realized I had been struggling for a while. I'd had several recent encounters at local shops with people who would greet me warmly and would speak intimately about my family and theirs. I knew I was supposed to know who they were, *but I didn't.* I fumbled my way through those conversations, trying to get away as quickly as possible. I had an episode when I was driving home from work on my regular route. I looked up at a stoplight near my home, and for a few terrifying seconds, I had no idea where I was. That feeling would occasionally reoccur without warning. It worried me enough that I began to plan my routes out, even to familiar places. Over time, my world became smaller and smaller.

I noticed that my personality was changing. My whole life, I'd been quick-witted, curious, upbeat, and hardworking. Now I had a hard time keeping up with conversations. I'd also been a voracious reader, but I was having a hard time remembering the characters, the plot, even the sentence I'd just read. Reading for pleasure was no longer pleasurable. Simple things that had once been easy—like balancing my checkbook, paying bills, or calculating a tip at a restaurant—became difficult. I couldn't understand why I was struggling with basic tasks. My husband and son commented on my short temper. They began to tiptoe around me, trying not to upset me. I saw the looks they exchanged, but I felt helpless to fix things.

Until then, I had thought of death as something that would happen in the distant future of some unknown cause. If I truly had Alzheimer's, I had met my enemy face-to-face. I realized that I could be slipping into what's been poignantly described as the "long goodbye." Coincidentally, one of the last novels that I'd read was *Still Alice,* in which a woman with early-onset Alzheimer's makes a plan to kill herself, but later forgets and is unable to carry it out. I considered the idea myself, but my plan was to do it *earlier, before I would forget.* To die by losing the essence of myself and putting my family through the burden of caring for me was unbearable. If I killed myself, at least I'd die with dignity on my own terms. At the same time, a thought kept growing stronger inside me: *What if the doctors were wrong? What if there was something I could do to turn this around?*

I felt an almost animal-like instinct to move back to where

I'd grown up, on the shores of Lake Michigan. A perfect place to die . . . *or fight*. I wasn't sure which one yet. I wanted to be near my family. Because I carried two copies of this gene, I knew that other members of my family were also at an increased risk. The timing was perfect, since our son was heading off to college. My husband and I left the wonderful life that we'd created for ourselves in the foothills of the North Georgia mountains and we moved to northwestern Indiana. We moved into a tiny condo on a small lake just a few blocks from Lake Michigan.

I recall an incident that occurred while we were on a house-hunting trip. My son was confused and angry with us for leaving our beautiful home, our friends, and everything familiar. He couldn't understand why we were making this move. I finally told him everything. I told him about my high genetic risk for Alzheimer's, how I was already exhibiting symptoms, my fear that I was dying. My strong, independent, six-foot-one man-child broke down into tears. We held each other and both sobbed. He said, *"Mom, I don't want you to die."*

From that moment on, I knew I had to fight. I had to be there for my son. I wanted to meet his future wife and their children. This was the motivation I needed. *I chose to live.*

LOST IN A MEDICAL MAZE

Before I outline the steps that ultimately led to my recovery, I want to touch upon the many strange and seemingly unrelated medical symptoms that I'd experienced up to this point. In hindsight, I now realize that many either directly contributed to or were a result of the underlying drivers of my cognitive decline.

Hypoglycemia (low blood sugar), which I experienced off and on throughout my adulthood, dramatically worsened in the years preceding my time of reckoning. I almost lost consciousness twice. I was forced to eat more and more often just to maintain stability. In retrospect, I was certainly insulin resistant. Those blood sugar lows were almost certainly preceded by high swings. For the first time in my life, my weight slowly crept up to 20 pounds above my baseline, primarily in my abdomen, while my blood pressure also trended upward to an average of 140/90.

During this period, I also began to suffer from debilitating night sweats and extreme allergy symptoms that even led to full-blown anaphylaxis, a life-threatening allergic reaction. I would develop itchy skin, hive-like rashes, flushing, sneezing attacks, throat and chest constriction that left me gasping for air, accompanied by tachycardia (rapid heartbeat); all reversed by my EpiPen. My allergist did extensive testing, which revealed that I was allergic to absolutely *nothing*. He suspected mast cell activation syndrome (MCAS, a malfunction of the immune system), later confirmed at Brigham and Women's Hospital, and put me on massive doses of antihistamines. Although the treatment likely saved my life, I retrospectively understand that antihistamines, because of their anticholinergic properties, which block the action of acetylcholine necessary for learning and memory, have been correlated with the development of dementia.

I'd also been experiencing worsening blood circulation issues. This began in my early 30s, shortly after my son was born—my hands and feet were almost always cold and became covered in small sores. I was diagnosed with Raynaud's syndrome and put on a blood pressure medication to dilate my blood vessels and improve my circulation. That initially alleviated the symptoms, but my blood pressure dropped so low that I was too fatigued to function. I eventually switched to a daily low-dose aspirin, but my Raynaud's symptoms continued to wax and wane, escalating at times to cyanotic extremities (blue fingers and toes) that required multiple hospitalizations.

Underlying this picture were my ongoing gastrointestinal (GI) and bladder issues. The GI symptoms first showed up when I was in my early 20s. Following almost every meal, I would experience severe lower abdominal pain and diarrhea. One time, in my late 20s, I began to experience a different type of pain, this time in my upper abdomen, pain so severe I was unable to eat or even drink water. I was told my liver enzymes were extremely elevated, but I was negative for hepatitis. I was hospitalized for weeks with an IV drip and morphine for pain without ever receiving a definitive diagnosis.

During my 40s, the upper abdominal pain recurred with a vengeance. The doctors determined that my gallbladder had stopped working, and it was finally removed. My surgeon noted that my gallbladder was wrapped in layers of adhesions, indicating that it may have ruptured decades earlier. However, rather than providing relief, I became even *sicker* after that surgery. My GI motility completely stopped, and my blood pressure tanked. I was unable to eat or even stand up. I ended up back in the hospital and was ultimately rescued with medication to raise my blood pressure and instructed to use mega-doses of MiraLAX, polyethylene glycol, as a laxative, which I later learned is quite toxic.

Starting in my mid-20s, I experienced my first bladder infection. It was extraordinarily severe and wouldn't resolve. I was ultimately put on *years* of antibiotics, despite a negative bladder culture, because a cystoscopy revealed my bladder was so inflamed that my urologist described it as having appearance of "red velvet" and remarked that he'd never seen anything like it. Despite that treatment, I continued to experience severe bladder pain and a sense of urgency that lingered for years.

Compounding these multiple chronic health issues was the trauma that resulted from a vehicle collision in my early 30s. I was briefly unconscious and suffered severe head pain and whiplash, which left me with persistent pain for over a decade. My neurologist eventually put me on amitriptyline, an antidepressant, to help with the chronic pain. It is *another* anticholinergic medication that is contraindicated for anyone at high risk of Alzheimer's.

In my late 40s, I was diagnosed with a large symptomatic uterine fibroid. I opted for a uterine fibroid embolization, in which a radiologist injects small particles into the arteries leading to the fibroid tumor, causing it to shrink over time. My fibroid ultimately did shrink, but the blood supply to my ovaries was damaged, leading to an abrupt onset of menopause, which can also contribute to cognitive decline. Eleven years later, I still had to have a hysterectomy and pelvic reconstruction as a result of an underlying familial connective tissue disorder, first evidenced by a hernia repair at age five.

In horrifying retrospect, without ever knowing I was genetically fragile, I had unwittingly undergone multiple rounds of general anesthesia and had taken many medications (massive amounts of antibiotics, anticholinergics, and toxic amounts of polyethylene glycol) that in the short term helped my symptoms but could potentially have harmed my cognition.

Despite all of this, I continued to put on a brave front to the outside world. I never identified myself as being "sick." Few people were even aware of my health struggles. Once I learned of my high genetic risk for Alzheimer's, after everyone in my family had fallen asleep, I'd quietly google into the wee hours, trying to figure out if my medical symptoms could be related. None of the conventional literature that I'd found made such a link. Alzheimer's was always described as affecting the brain only, as if the brain were disconnected from the body? That made no sense to me.

Fortunately, 23andMe provided forums where folks could gather to discuss what they'd learned in their genetic results. I eventually found my way to the Alzheimer's forum, and in doing so, I found my lifeline, my new surrogate family. People from all over the world were also learning of their high genetic risk and struggling with the information. *I no longer felt alone.*

Not only did my newly discovered ApoE4 tribe offer vital emotional support but we also became deeply immersed in the science. We wanted to learn everything we could about our high-risk gene in an effort to find strategies that could prevent, mitigate, or delay the onset of Alzheimer's. I voraciously read every new journal article or scientific study I could find, often with a medical dictionary nearby, trying to make sense of what I was reading. Over time, our group amassed an impressive collection of ApoE4-related information. In 2013, I worked with a small team to move our discussions to our own website, called ApoE4.Info, where we could better organize and catalog our work. Shortly afterward, we attained nonprofit status for our project, where we continue to interact with researchers from all over the world and run an online community, a Facebook page, and a wiki, where we support and educate those with ApoE4 while searching for answers to mitigate its pathological effects.

It's important to remember that back in 2012, the medical community lacked a consensus about what, if any, strategies ApoE4 carriers should adopt to protect themselves, with one exception: a very low-fat diet was strongly recommended to protect against heart disease, and by default, Alzheimer's. At that time, the orthodox scientific theory for Alzheimer's was the amyloid hypothesis, which posited that the disease was caused by a buildup of malformed protein in the brain. Researchers back then often associated high cholesterol with a higher burden of both cardiovascular disease and beta-amyloid plaques found in the brains of those who died with Alzheimer's. However, another hypothesis was emerging that suggested Alzheimer's was really "type 3 diabetes," because patients with prediabetes and diabetes appeared to be at higher risk for the disease.

Members of our community were evenly and passionately divided. Those who leaned toward the amyloid hypothesis tended to eat a low-fat, high-carbohydrate diet, whereas those who leaned toward the alternate hypothesis ate a high-fat, low-carbohydrate diet. We had no idea which theory would prevail. We were literally modern-day canaries in the coal mine, gambling with our lives.

I wanted to enlist the help of a neurologist and sought out the most esteemed physician in my area. I told him about my high genetic risk and the symptoms I'd been experiencing. I asked him what I could do to prevent them from worsening, or better, to reverse them. His response: "Good luck with that." No offer to do cognitive testing, imaging—nothing. He dismissed the possible lifestyle and diet strategies that I brought up. I was devastated. I later learned that many members of our ApoE4.Info community had had similar experiences. One of our members reported that his neurologist actually said: "Go home and wait for it."

FINDING MY WAY BACK

Around this time, I found a lecture on the internet, given by Dr. David Perlmutter. He immediately had my attention with the title "Alzheimer's CAN Be Prevented." I listened to that lecture many times. I took avid notes, especially on his supplement recommendations. He was a practicing neurologist in Naples, Florida. I decided to visit him, but I had to wait several months before I could get an appointment.

In the meantime, my own healing journey was well under way. As I learned about potentially helpful strategies with my ApoE4 tribe, I began to apply them. I started with exercise and began to view it in a different way. Instead of pushing myself with boot-camp-style workouts, I began to look at exercise as "my time," a one-hour (or longer) daily opportunity to nurture myself. I walked outside every day. I sometimes listened to meditative music, sometimes to music that just made me happy. The Rolling Stones and Neil Young serenaded me as I trekked along Lake Shore Drive, mesmerized by the beauty and power of Lake Michigan. I would occasionally journey back to my childhood neighborhood, about a seven-mile round trip. I had returned to my homeplace to die, but instead was finding strength in my roots.

I changed my diet, starting by cutting out all sugar. I reduced processed and refined foods. As I learned about omega-3s and omega-6s, I worked to balance them, increasing omega-3s. I began adding some fermented food into my diet. I decided to try some targeted supplements. The first was curcumin, an extract from turmeric. It took three tries, but I finally found a brand that didn't cause a mast cell reaction called Terry Naturally CuraMed. Within a day or two, I began to experience a lifting and lightening of my mood. Widespread body pain that had been present for years markedly abated. I had more energy. I began adding other supplements. Some like acetyl-L-carnitine, alpha-lipoic acid, and N-acetyl cysteine I learned about from Dr. Perlmutter's lecture. Others he recommended, like fish oil and vitamin D, I had already learned about from papers I had read.

Understanding that my high-risk genotype poorly eliminates heavy metals and toxins, I found aluminum-free sunscreen and antiperspirant and found alternatives for many of my toiletries and cosmetics that contained toxic chemicals. I stopped using nail polish and instead switched to using coconut oil on my cuticles, fingernails, and toenails. I stopped using mouthwash when I became aware that, in addition to killing harmful bacteria, mouthwash also destroyed good bacteria. And for the first time, I began to meditate. I found amazing freedom in turning my mind inward, leading to a sense of calm that extended beyond my meditation sessions.

By the time I got to see Dr. Perlmutter in Florida, I was already much improved. My husband accompanied me to my long-awaited appointment. There was a night and day difference from the experience I'd had with my local neurologist. Dr. Perlmutter did cognitive testing, ran some blood work, and reviewed an old MRI that I had brought with me. He strongly encouraged me to adopt a grain-free, low-carb Paleo diet, consisting of clean, whole foods. He also recommended a few additional supplements based upon my blood-work results. I knew that a Paleo diet was quite high in fat, which felt unsettling to me at that time. Through experimentation, our ApoE4 community was learning that we had a hyper-response to dietary fat, especially saturated fat. It took a while before I was fully ready to integrate that facet of his recommendation into my approach.

Nevertheless, both my husband and I were inspired to change our diet pretty radically after meeting with Dr. Perlmutter. When we returned home, we began ruthlessly purging our well-stocked kitchen. Almost nothing remained at the end except for a bunch of (likely expired) spices and a few vegetables. I needed to figure out this new way of eating pretty quickly or we would starve! Learning how to source "clean" food in my small town was a challenge. I was stunned by the limited availability of organic produce at my local grocery stores. Because it was more expensive, it often sat on store shelves until it wilted, leaving me with a very small selection. I quickly learned which day it was delivered at each store, and made my rounds gathering local organic greens, colorful cruciferous vegetables, and fresh herbs.

I struggled to find clean animal protein. Everything I was learning suggested that animal protein from CAFOs (concentrated animal feeding operations) was suboptimal and even harmful. In an effort to increase profit, CAFOs house animals in very crowded quarters under stressful living conditions, leading them to become sick and in need of antibiotics. Indeed, most commercial operations prophylactically give antibiotics to prevent infections. These animals are fed unnatural grain-based diets, with growth hormones, encouraging quick maturation and weight gain. I learned that the effects of the antibiotics and growth hormones are passed along to us, as well as the inflammatory effects of the grains the animals eat. Finding 100 percent wild-caught seafood and pastured beef and poultry wasn't easy in my small town, but I ultimately found like-minded rebel citizens trying to eat the same way we were. As we learned about various co-ops, farmers' markets, and direct-to-consumer farm drop-off points, my husband and I would pack up our coolers to gather seasonal organic local produce, freshly laid eggs from pastured hens, and 100 percent grass-fed meat. We learned that Sam's Club (about a two-hour round trip) regularly stocked flash-frozen wild-caught seafood.

I was still dealing with occasional bouts of hypoglycemia. I figured if my body was struggling with a fuel deficit, there was a high likelihood that my brain was as well. I had been reading about experimental work using ketones to overcome this deficit. I decided to experiment on myself. Using urinary ketone strips (which are somewhat useful), I began actively working to reach ketosis. I began extending my daily fast a bit longer each day, exercising for longer periods, and increasing my dietary fat. All of these strategies finally turned the urine strips a lovely shade of pink, indicating that I was in ketosis. Over time, this completely resolved my hypoglycemia, and my cognition took a dramatic turn for the better.

With all of these strategies I was applying, my chronic and complex medical issues began to fade away. I no longer failed to remember people I should have known. I felt confident driving again. I was reading once more. In fact, I left behind the novels I'd previously enjoyed and was reading scientific and medical journal articles instead. I became passionate to learn everything I could about my ApoE4 gene: how it led to disease, and how I could intervene.

It was at this point, in September of 2014, that a member of our ApoE4.Info community posted a link to Dr. Bredesen's paper, "Reversal of Cognitive Decline: A Novel Therapeutic Program." This astounding article described improvement in nine out of ten people in individual case studies and detailed the scientific theory behind that success. It outlined specific programs that these patients had used to *reverse* cognitive decline. I was well aware that no other Alzheimer's researcher had ever made such a brash claim. My heart began to beat more quickly as I read the case studies. *These people were using strategies very similar to those I had been employing for the last several years to heal from my own cognitive decline.* Tears of joy ran down my face.

I decided to reach out to Dr. Bredesen with an email. I wanted to share my story with him, to let him know that his approach had helped me, too. I was stunned when he wrote back and arranged a phone call. We spoke that same day. He asked lots of questions, and I could hear him taking notes. I told him about our community of ApoE4 carriers, many using a similar approach to prevent and remediate symptoms of cognitive decline. He was delighted to learn of our community and our work. I was struck by both his kindness and his curiosity.

Dr. Bredesen offered to look over my biomarkers and made a few suggestions. He proposed that I try herbal supplements like ashwagandha (sometimes called Indian ginseng) to help deal with stress and improve sleep. He also proposed that I work on increasing my estrogen level through bioidentical hormones, as it was quite low at the time. Both changes had positive effects.

Several months later, in May of 2015, members of our ApoE4 .Info community held our first meet-up in San Francisco. Our event kicked off with a visit to the Buck Institute for Research on Aging, which Dr. Bredesen had helped to found. Despite the fact we had never met the other members in person before, it felt like a family reunion. We were given a guided tour of the institute's magnificent I. M. Pei–designed building. My favorite part was visiting Dr. Bredesen's research lab; seeing his test tubes, petri dishes, and transgenic mice helped me to fully understand that his theory was born out of decades of hard-core laboratory research.

We were then ushered into the Drexler Auditorium, where a large crowd had gathered to hear Dr. Bredesen. He had asked me to speak first, to describe my journey. My knees were weak; I had never done any public speaking before. It felt like everyone held a collective breath as I began to share my story. I could see the effect my words were having on the audience. Some hugged loved ones sitting next to them. I realized that I wasn't the only one who had been through this. I ended by saying, "It's my honor to introduce the man who offers *hope*, Dr. Dale Bredesen. That is what he did for me and for countless others in an environment that otherwise offered nothing but despair."

After this meeting, Dr. Bredesen often called to share new findings from his research and lab. Unlike any other Alzheimer's researcher I communicated with, he also wanted to know what we were working on. I shared my excitement about the additional cognitive improvements I was experiencing by utilizing my version of a mildly ketogenic approach. I could sense his skepticism. The Paleo diet, recommended by Dr. Perlmutter and trending back then, is high in animal protein and saturated fat, basically the opposite of Dr. Bredesen's heavily plant-based approach. I had merged the two in a way that was proving helpful for me and for others in my community. I replaced foods like bacon, butter, and coconut oil—high in saturated fat that had a negative effect on my lipid profile—with fatty fish, extra-virgin olive oil, avocados, nuts, and seeds, high in monounsaturated and polyunsaturated fats, instead. By combining this modified version of the diet with a longer daily fast and exercise, I and other members of our community were endogenously creating a mild level of ketosis that provided a noticeable cognitive boost and steady energy, while yielding excellent glycemic *and* lipid biomarkers. I continued to bring it up every time we spoke. Dr. Bredesen ended one memorable phone call with: "Hey, I think you're onto something." *I knew I was.*

Dr. Bredesen kindly reached out to me prior to the publication of two important papers to share what he'd uncovered. The first, published in September of 2015, described three distinct subtypes of Alzheimer's (now recognized as six subtypes). Several months later, Dr. Bredesen contacted me to share a new finding. Toxins from molds were, surprisingly, turning out to be a frequent contributor to Alzheimer's disease, as they are to chronic inflammatory response syndrome (CIRS). CIRS is a condition in which some patients exposed to toxins, often biotoxins like mold toxins or those from a tick bite, became chronically ill. The many varied symptoms sounded a lot like mast cell activation syndrome, which I, and a surprising number of others in my ApoE4 community, had experienced.

At this point I had begun to experience a plateau in my healing. Traveling was hard on me. If I deviated at all from my diet or skimped on sleep, I really felt the effects. I began having significant issues maintaining my body temperature, uncontrollably shivering even in warm weather. I wasn't handling stress well. Most frightening, I felt my cognition slipping. Dr. Bredesen pushed me to test for CIRS. I would occasionally see him at various conferences or meetings. Once as I passed him in a stairwell, he called out: "What's your TGF-beta-1? How about C4a? Do you know your MSH?" I felt slightly harassed. I had no idea what he was talking about.

Because of Dr. Bredesen's repeated urging, however, I finally engaged in some testing. Of course, he was spot-on. Every single one of my preliminary CIRS tests was horribly out of range. One of the tests he'd encouraged me to take was the HLA DR/DQ haplotype, a kind of genetic signature that reveals a susceptibility to a specific biotoxin. My results indicated I was susceptible to a chronic Lyme infection. *Lyme disease?* Thinking back, I had experienced tick bites throughout my life. Growing up with three brothers, I was a tomboy. Rolling in the dirt, building forts in the woods, and running through the dune grass at the beach were all commonplace activities. Once in my early 40s, however, I had a different kind of tick bite. By the time I discovered it, it had the telltale bull's-eye Lyme rash around it. My physician put me on a weeklong round of antibiotics, which seemed to do the trick, but maybe the dose was not strong or long enough.

Dr. Bredesen helped me get an appointment with Dr. Sunjya Schweig at the California Center for Functional Medicine. All of my Lyme testing turned out to be negative, but I was overwhelmingly positive (very high antibody titers) for a Lyme disease co-infection called *Babesia duncani*. As I learned more about my form of babesiosis, I realized that it likely had been responsible for many of my ongoing chronic health issues and may have even been the primary driver behind my cognitive decline. *Babesia duncani* is a malaria-like infection of the red blood cells. Sometimes the cells are enlarged and have difficulty getting through the capillaries, perhaps contributing to my cyanotic digits. Air hunger, temperature dysregulation, and even tachycardia are common symptoms. Another common symptom is cognitive decline. In many ways, I was a classic case of babesiosis, *but none of my physicians had ever considered this.*

Dr. Schweig was able to skip through many of his typical initial recommendations for healing—diet, exercise, sleep optimization, stress management, etc.—because I had already begun applying them. He put me on an antimicrobial regimen, a twice-daily targeted babesiosis herbal infusion, and recommended intravenous immunoglobulin (IVIG) replacement therapy to bolster my immune system to address my worsening hypogammaglobulinemia (low IgG). He theorized that my immune system had become so overwhelmed by the babesiosis that it was "burnt out." It was scary the first time I got the IVIG therapy at my local cancer care center, as anaphylaxis (which I'd previously experienced) is a possible side effect. I was hooked up to an IV for an infusion that lasted almost four hours. But I felt fine the next morning, maybe even *better than fine*. I went out for my hourlong trek, and for the first time in a long time, I had to run. I felt so energized that I couldn't simply walk. That extreme benefit lasted several days following the infusion and suggested to me that it was having a positive effect.

MY DAILY PROTOCOL

Please keep in mind that I've been using this approach for eight years, since before it was a "thing," and my strategies have evolved over time. What I do today is nothing like what I did at the beginning. I took baby steps to get where I am now. Also, given my history and very high genetic risk, I try pretty hard. I'm a bit of a geek and enjoy the science, trying out new strategies that lead to steady tweaks of my protocol. Also, it's important to understand that every protocol is unique, based upon specific risks and contributors. It's most important to identify whatever may be driving any potential pathology and specifically prioritize that.

- I wake up between five and six A.M., without an alarm, after seven to eight hours of sleep. I've gotten into a very ancestral circadian rhythm, where I go to bed with the sunset and wake up with the sunrise. I love my mornings and wake up full of energy and purpose to take on the new day.

- Upon awakening, I take fifteen minutes to meditate. This practice provides a sense of centered awareness that helps me make mindful choices throughout the day.

- I skip breakfast and enjoy a cup or two of mold-free organic coffee (note that some coffee beans include molds and the mycotoxins they produce), no cream or sugar, with a very small amount of stevia. I'm very careful to stop all beverages containing caffeine early in the day, typically before nine A.M. If I cheat with an early afternoon cup of coffee as a pick-me-up, my sleep is definitely affected.

- To protect the enamel on my teeth from the acidity of my coffee, as soon as I have finished drinking it, I rinse (swish) my teeth with water before gently brushing them with a non-fluoride toothpaste.

- I also use aluminum-free sunscreen and deodorant. I always consult the Environmental Working Group's Skin Deep database to find the safest toiletries and cosmetics.

- I then head outside almost every single day, regardless of the weather, and enjoy at least a 3.5-mile walk or run. This is my favorite part of the day. I find spending time in nature to be very healing. I love seeing the seasons and the wildlife, and feeling the weather on my skin. I still live near the shores of Lake Michigan and experience tremendous weather extremes, from wind gales that make it difficult to walk to temperatures well below zero. This is a way for me to practice hormesis—the theory that regular exposure to adversity builds strength.

- I like to combine strategies, and sometimes I listen to educational podcasts or take an online class as I'm exercising. Other times, I listen to my favorite music to energize me or to meditative music if I need to problem-solve. I also love letting my mind wander while listening to nature.

- Upon returning home, I'll shower with nontoxic castile soap if I'm sweaty. Several times a week, I hop in my low-EMF portable sauna before showering to aid in additional detoxification and to create shock proteins that repair damaged proteins in my body and help to heal oxidative damage prior to showering.

- I then prepare a big glass of room-temperature matcha tea (high in neuroprotective epigallocatechin gallate) with silica water (which helps to chelate aluminum) and put all of my morning supplements, those I've found to be energizing, in a little ramekin and head up to my office to begin my day of work. It's much less daunting to swallow supplements when I do it slowly, sometimes over an hour, while I'm working. If it feels difficult to swallow them, I sometimes casually walk around the house or even begin slowly cycling on my stationary bike while taking my supplements. Simply moving, even slowly, helps me to more easily swallow and digest the supplements. See my full morning list below.

> - DHA, 1000 mg
> - Cod-liver oil, ½ tsp
> - Plasmalogen supplement
> - Curcumin (BCM-95), 750 mg
> - Vitamin E (mixed tocotrienols 145 mg and tocopherols 360 mg)
> - Vitamin D3, 6000 IU
> - Vitamin K1 and K2 (Life Extension, Super K), 1 capsule
> - Methylcobalamin, 1 mg
> - Folate (Metafolin), 800 mcg
> - Pyrroloquinoline quinone, 20 mg
> - Pyridoxal-5'-phosphate, 20 mg
> - N-acetyl cysteine, 600 mg
> - Alpha-lipoic acid, 225 mg
> - Acetyl-L-carnitine, 525 mg
> - Ubiquinol, 200 mg
> - Lecithin (phosphatidylcholine), 333 mg
> - Kinoko Platinum AHCC, 750 mg
> - Resveratrol (Longevinex blend), 335 mg
> - Nicotinamide riboside, 100 mg

> MegaSporeBiotic, 1 capsule
> Dr. Shade's Bitters no. 9, two pumps after a meal if my stomach feels overly full

• As I work, I make a point of walking around for ten to fifteen minutes of every hour. Because I work from home, this is a great opportunity to do household chores, which I've learned to reframe as "exercise opportunities."

• I alternate between a sixteen-hour and a twenty-hour fast, typically eating one meal a day, sometimes two. I realize that this feels extreme to many people. Keep in mind that it took me a long time to get to this point. When I first began the protocol, I was insulin resistant and often awoke with hypoglycemia in the middle of the night and had to eat a snack. I took baby steps to heal my metabolism, which enabled my body to be able to get into ketosis, so I can now easily fast for a long period of time.

• My ketones are often at their highest point of the day (typically between 1 and 2 mM) right before I break my fast. I sometimes check my ketones, but rarely check my glucose at this point in my recovery. My Hba1c has been steady between 4.7 and 4.8 for years, and while regular glucose and ketone checks as well as journaling my food intake with an online food diary called Cronometer (cronometer .com) was very helpful in the beginning, I no longer need that level of detailed tracking.

- Prior to breaking my fast, I drink a glass of water with lemon and/or ginger to detoxify, and I take two glucosamine chondroitin capsules to help with lectin sensitivity. (Lectins, such as gluten, are sticky plant proteins that can cause inflammation for those who are sensitive.) Even though I generally eat a grain-free, low-lectin diet, I concurrently use the glucosamine chondroitin to help block the effects of lectins still remaining from vegetables in my diet.

- If I eat two meals, which I do when I notice a downward trend in my weight, my first meal would be enjoyed after noon and would typically include two pastured eggs with a plateful of organic non-starchy vegetables, comprised of leafy greens and cruciferous and colorful vegetables (some raw, some cooked), including prebiotic fiber like jicama, mushrooms, or scallions along with a small amount of resistant starch such as a few cooked and cooled sweet potato wedges along with a few tablespoons of fermented vegetables. I finish my vegetables with liberal amounts (several tablespoons) of high-polyphenol extra-virgin olive oil, with fresh herbs and spices, along with Himalayan sea salt and dried sea vegetables for iodine.

- After each meal, I carefully floss and gently brush with a non-fluoride toothpaste. Because there is a strong link between oral and brain health, I also have my teeth professionally cleaned three times a year as opposed to twice, even though I don't have any ongoing periodontal or other issues.

- A few times a week, I drink a cup of grass-fed bone broth for its gut-healing benefits along with a meal.

- Between five and seven days a week, I engage in a thirty-minute KAATSU strength-training program. This is a therapeutic Japanese practice that mildly restricts blood flow to the arms and legs and tricks my muscles into thinking they're working much harder than they're actually working. The benefit is twofold. One, I'm increasing my muscle strength without actually breaking down muscle fiber. This is a huge benefit for everyone, but especially for those who are middle-aged and older. Second, by creating this mild hypoxic state in my muscles, I'm upregulating many healing growth hormones like BDNF and plasmalogens, that also have neuroprotective benefits.

- After exercise or sauna and throughout the day, I'm careful to stay hydrated. I sip room-temperature filtered water or S.Pellegrino as a refreshing way to replenish minerals. As mentioned earlier, I also use sea salt to avoid keto flu (flu-like symptoms that sometimes appear with ketosis, often due to fluid loss) and maintain fluid balance. Staying well hydrated promotes optimal detoxification.

- I usually take a midafternoon break from work and challenge myself to a twenty-minute brain-training session using BrainHQ or another brain-training site. I'm currently experimenting with Elevate and like that the exercises translate into tangible improvements in my real-life performance.

• Afterward, I like to meditate for another fifteen-minute session. I'm not always faithful to this second session, but I feel so much better when I can squeeze it in. Regular practice has tremendous mood, energy, and sleep benefits.

• I eat my second meal between four and five P.M. or a bit earlier, two to three P.M., if I'm eating just one meal. If my husband is home, we make this main meal a time of celebration. We've typically been apart, focused on our own schedules, and this is our chance to reconnect and nurture with food. We often plan our menu over coffee in the morning and cook together. A typical meal might include wild-caught fish, such as Alaskan sockeye salmon, with a large colorful salad consisting of a variety of equally colorful, non-starchy, high-fiber organic vegetables (some cooked, some raw) dressed liberally with high-polyphenol EVOO, lots of fresh herbs and spices, Himalayan sea salt, and dried sea vegetables for iodine. If this is our only meal of the day, we typically alternate between pastured eggs or low-mercury, wild-caught seafood as the protein. We always include a little bit of resistant starch, prebiotic fiber, and fermented veggies on our plates.

• I refrain from snacking between meals, but if I'm eating only one main meal (sticking to a four-hour eating window), I freely nibble as I cook and even snack an hour or so afterward. This helps me maintain my weight without gorging myself at one sitting.

- As a rare treat, I sometimes sip two to three ounces of dry sugar-free low-alcohol organic red wine after my main meal.

- I occasionally enjoy dessert during my eating window. One of my favorites is raw organic walnuts, julienned almonds, coconut flakes, and wild berries drizzled with sugar-free nut or goat milk. Another treat would be a carefully chosen (low cadmium and lead) dark chocolate square or two, 86 percent or higher cacao.

- I stop eating by six P.M. (often much earlier) and put on my blue blocking glasses if I'm still using screens or artificial light. I prefer to dim the lights during this wind-down period and try to refrain from stimulating work or conversations.

- I like to take my evening supplements an hour or so before bed with just enough water to safely swallow them so I can avoid bathroom runs in the middle of the night. You can see a full list of my evening supplements and medications, those I've found to have a sedating effect, below.
  - > Magnesium glycinate, 1500 mg
  - > Melatonin, 3 mg
  - > Ashwagandha, 300 mg

> GABA (gamma-aminobutryic acid), 500 mg
> Transdermal estradiol patch, 0.1 mg per day, changed midweek
> Progesterone, 100 mg
> Testosterone gel, 1 to 2 drops applied on forearm every other evening
> Sunfiber prebiotic, 1 scoop
> Schiff Digestive Advantage, 1 capsule
> Low-dose naltrexone, 3 mg

• Every two months, I continue to require IVIG infusion to keep my IgG within the normal reference range, albeit near the bottom. After several years of treatment, I'm babesiosis-free and have been able to drop both the dosage and frequency of my IVIG therapy. My hope is that as my immune system heals, this will no longer be necessary.

• Before bed, using dim blue-blocking light, I gently wash my face with a nontoxic cleanser and use the Ayurvedic practice of oil pulling with coconut oil, which has antimicrobial properties. I just melt one to two teaspoons of coconut oil in my mouth and pull it through and around my teeth for fifteen minutes. I find this very relaxing, and (I don't understand why) it also helps me to sleep much more deeply.

• I like to get into bed (not necessarily to sleep) by eight P.M. During this wind-down period, my husband and I often run some additional passive KAATSU sets with our automated pneumatic systems. The bands inflate and deflate themselves while we're relaxing and reading in bed. I sometimes unconsciously engage in gentle isometric exercises during this time. I notice that running through several KAATSU cycles before bed helps me to quickly fall asleep and sleep more deeply.

- I use this time to read pleasurable fiction using the Kindle app on my iPad with the brightness set to the lowest setting and Night Shift enabled to block blue light. I also turn the lights off and keep our room completely darkened. Any small amount of light can interfere with melatonin production. I've also selected my iPad to automatically turn itself off if I stop moving for five minutes. This often allows me to gently fall asleep without having to turn off the bedside lamp.

- Additionally, I sleep on a (non-EMF) cooling mattress pad, set to 65 degrees, which helps me fall asleep quickly, as a lower core body temperature also helps to boost melatonin production. And, because I sometimes toss and turn as I fall asleep, I cover myself with a weighted blanket, which almost instantly provides a sense of calm that helps me to drift off.

I rarely carry out my own protocol perfectly. I just do the best I can. Like everyone, I'm faced with dozens of decisions throughout each day, I'm fully aware that some move me toward health, while others move me away from health. As I encounter these forks in the road, I recall a stark yet poignant quote from *The Shawshank Redemption* that beautifully summarizes the ultimate consequence of my choices and helps keep me on track: "Get busy living or get busy dying." I do my best to consciously choose life every single day. The benefits have been enormous, rendering my way of life quite sustainable for me.

Rather than feeling bitter that I suffered for so many years without answers, I feel blessed to have them now. Perhaps because I keenly remember my darkest days on this journey, I see every day as a gift.

My cognitive testing scores have risen dramatically; from the mid-30th percentile to the high-90th percentile for my age group. However, what surprised me the most was that many of my previous health issues have either completely disappeared or greatly improved. I now feel healthier and stronger—with calm, steady energy throughout the day—than at any other point in my adult life. It took Dr. Bredesen's keen insight to identify what was likely the primary driver of my cognitive decline and my many seemingly disconnected medical symptoms. That knowledge has provided vital information enabling me to embark upon a targeted healing journey that continues to this day.

I know that my transformation wouldn't have been possible without my husband, Bruce. He's not only walked beside me in terms of offering support, but he's also adopted the vast majority of my diet and lifestyle changes . . . *and benefited greatly.* He's lost 30 pounds, traded his spare tire for muscle, and no longer takes any prescription medicine. As an international airline pilot, who often chooses to fast during long transoceanic flights, he's stunned by the poor attention and stamina of his younger copilots, who rely on carbohydrates for fuel. In turn, they can't believe he's so full of energy. Many have begun to ask for health tips and have ultimately chosen to adopt his approach. In fact, at a recent semiannual FAA-required physical, his physician asked him to reveal his secret to aging backward. For spouses who are on the fence about adopting the protocol, I promise it won't hurt you, and I have no doubt that much of my success lies in the fact that we've made this "our lifestyle" as opposed to "my treatment."

My son, who once begged me not to die, has since graduated from college. He unexpectedly chose to follow in his father's footsteps and has become an airline pilot. I've survived long enough to meet his wife and dance at their wedding. My husband and I have since moved from our tiny condo, where I once prepared for my final chapter, deeper into our beloved neighborhood still on the same beautiful lake, where we've renovated a neglected older home with lots of room for our future grandchildren. We often walk hand in hand through our neighborhood, relishing our bonus years, which were almost lost.

You might have seen that TV commercial where the Alzheimer's Association searches for the first survivor, so they can present him or her with a special white flower. Keep your rare bloom. Give me weeds and wildflowers, with deep roots, that break through the toughest soil and survive the harshest conditions—thriving where they shouldn't—with an unappreciated, tenacious beauty recognized only by those willing to look beyond the expected.

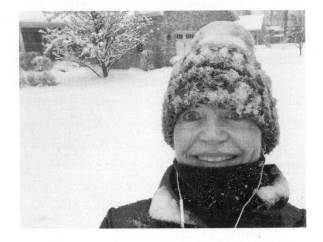

COMMENT: Julie's remarkable journey reinforces the point that cognitive decline is a response to insults, which are typically multiple and often systemic: her babesiosis, multiple infections, many courses of antibiotics, glucose abnormalities, multiple administrations of anesthetics, anticholinergics, antihistamines, and rapid induction of menopause all likely contributed to her cognitive decline—which, especially in the setting of two copies of the pro-inflammatory ApoE4, are inducers of Alzheimer's-associated changes.

Addressing these contributors, largely by rectifying the genetic mismatch between her ancestral ApoE4 allele and the accumulation of modern insults, has led to her improvement, which has been sustained and even enhanced. Indeed, her story and those of the over 3,000 members of the ApoE4.Info community are living examples of the translation of our laboratory findings and resulting theory into real life. Julie has contributed her research with her community and her personal experience of living the protocol for over eight years to help us create the details of the program. I am deeply grateful for the work she has done, and the daily effort she shares with us to reduce the global burden of dementia.

Julie's story also illustrates beautifully two important lessons from the years of research and the many people now on the protocol. First, the era of hopelessness is over. Second, keep optimizing! It took Julie several years to address all of the many contributors to her cognitive decline, just as it did for Marcy. Therefore, no matter whether you respond initially or not, please keep tweaking to get the best results.

Now you have heard directly from seven different people—seven of hundreds—who experienced cognitive decline, and instead of simply slowing the decline, they actually *reversed* the decline. Furthermore, they *sustained* the improvement instead of returning to decline. They used a targeted, precision medicine approach to achieve the reversal.

We have recently published a paper describing a hundred patients who followed the same protocol, resulting in improvement that was documented and quantified in each one. In the following sections, this precise, systems approach to cognitive decline will be described in detail. I wish for each person the success that was realized by Kristin, Deborah, Edward, Marcy, Sally, Frank, Julie, and the hundreds of others like them.

On a final note, might it be possible to extrapolate the strategy utilized for these seven survivors to other diseases? This question will be addressed in chapter 11. Meanwhile, there is a critical need for a solution to the rare patient with familial Alzheimer's disease: about 95 percent of patients with Alzheimer's have sporadic Alzheimer's, which is the standard, in which there may be inherited risk—often from ApoE4—but there is no certainty that patients at risk for sporadic Alzheimer's will indeed develop it. In contrast, for that other 5 percent, the rare familial Alzheimer's, there is a direct inheritance of certainty, and no drug trial has ever affected the outcome in those patients. Since this is purely genetic, per-haps no intervention short of altering the gene itself will prove to be effective—but perhaps what we have learned to date can be extrapo-lated to help families with familial Alzheimer's disease.

Linda and her family members have such a mutation—a very rare mutation in APP itself, the amyloid precursor protein from which the am-yloid peptide is derived. Every one of her family members with the muta-tion develops Alzheimer's disease between 39 and 51 years of age, so as you can readily imagine, it has been very difficult for the children and siblings to watch one family member after another develop severe dementia.

There are over a hundred families in the world with APP mutations associated with Alzheimer's, and there has never been any result to sug-gest hope for these families. Linda's doctor was kind enough to put her in his car and drive her hundreds of miles to see me in 2013—so Linda is Patient Zero for familial Alzheimer's disease. Unfortunately, she already had a large amount of amyloid accumulation shown on her PET scan. However, her symptoms were still mild, and without any proven alterna-tive, she began on our protocol. She recently celebrated her 54th birth-day and had an extensive neuropsychological evaluation, showing no decline over the past eight years. How long can this delay in symptoms last? Might it have occurred just by chance? Only time will tell, but I hope that Linda will prove to be yet another of the Alzheimer's survivors.

PART TWO

Toward a World of Survivors

CHAPTER 8

Questions and Pushback: Resistance Training

The only way to avoid criticism is to
do nothing, say nothing, and be nothing.
—ARISTOTLE

As you might imagine, since our original medical paper on the reversal of cognitive decline was published in 2014, along with follow-ups in 2015, 2016, and 2018, many questions have been raised, clarifications requested, and concerns articulated, and much skepticism has been voiced about the results we have published. This is understandable—we are showing something in the publications that has never been shown before—and so skepticism is warranted. Therefore, I've responded, clarified, explained, and provided proof in this section, addressing some of the many questions and criticisms we have received.

- Does this approach help for other diseases, such as Parkinson's or Lewy body disease or Lou Gehrig's disease (ALS)?

We do not yet have enough data to determine whether this same approach will be effective for symptoms of neurodegenerative diseases other than Alzheimer's and its harbingers, MCI (mild cognitive impairment) and SCI (subjective cognitive impairment). Furthermore, the protocol would have to be modified to take into account the different underlying mechanisms for each disease, so it would not be identical to the ReCODE Protocol we have used for cognitive decline. Therefore, we have made the initial modifications, but to date have only a few anecdotal results. Thus, more work is needed to determine whether modified versions of the protocol will indeed be helpful for those with these other neurodegenerative conditions. However, we do have examples of Lewy body disease with documented improvement, and the evaluations of patients with Lewy body disease suggest that it is related to type 3 (toxic) Alzheimer's disease in that high levels of toxins (metallotoxins, organic toxins, or biotoxins) are typically present.

- **Aren't MCT oil and coconut oil saturated fats, and therefore particularly bad for people who carry the ApoE4 gene allele?**

People who are ApoE4-positive do have a higher risk for cardiovascular disease than those who are ApoE4-negative, and therefore saturated fat is a concern. However, MCT oil and coconut oil are very helpful for many who want to achieve ketosis, as well as for those wishing to avoid simple carbohydrates while needing energy. Therefore, there are two easy ways to get the best of both worlds—that is, improving brain energetics while avoiding vascular disease. First, you can use MCT oil or coconut oil for the first one to two months of the protocol in order to help support ketosis, then check your LDL-P (LDL particle number) and balance your MCT oil or coconut oil with unsaturated oils such as olive oil in order to keep your LDL-P below 1200 nM, while giving yourself the fats needed to continue ketosis. The second way is simply to use ketone salts or ketone esters to achieve ketosis, thus avoiding the saturated fat of MCT oil and coconut oil. In either case, the goal is to provide energy in the form of ketones, while minimizing simple carbohydrates like sugar, high-fructose corn syrup, and bread, and becoming insulin sensitive. In the long run, it is preferable to achieve endogenous ketosis (burning your own fat) instead of taking any form of exogenous ketones, but if this is not possible, then taking one of these forms of exogenous ketones can be very helpful.

- **How late in the course of Alzheimer's disease does the ReCODE Protocol work?**

As noted previously, we have seen a few people with MoCA (Montreal Cognitive Assessment Test) scores of 0—thus very late in the course—show improvement, but the later treatment is started, the less likely it is that improvement will occur, and in general the less complete the improvement will be. As a general rule, virtually all people with SCI who follow the protocol improve, most of those with MCI improve, and some of those with fully developed Alzheimer's improve.

Rosie is a 75-year-old woman with advanced Alzheimer's disease. She was unable to speak, unable to get up and walk, and unable to transfer herself from bed to chair. She began on the protocol, and after three months she was again speaking in sentences, interacting with her family and neighbor children, able to transfer herself from bed to chair, and able to get up and walk on her own.

• **Why does insurance usually not cover the testing and treatment?**

Although some insurance will cover all of the lab testing needed to determine the many contributors to cognitive decline for each person, it is true that unfortunately most insurance covers only a few of the tests. Similarly, for treatment, only partial coverage is typical. Something similar occurred for the first program to show reversal of cardiovascular disease, which was pioneered by Dr. Dean Ornish. Medicare took sixteen years to approve coverage of this successful and proven program. When Dean complained about this to a politician, the politician replied, "Only sixteen years?! How did you do get that done so quickly?!"

So the wheels of progress turn slowly, and I look forward to the day when insurance does indeed cover both the testing and the treatment. Since the cost of a nursing home far exceeds the cost of the protocol—the protocol is about 1 to 10 percent as costly as a nursing home, depending on which nursing home and the personal details of each person's protocol—then keeping anyone out of a nursing home for years (and hopefully for life) represents a major savings, one I hope insurance companies that provide long-term-care policies will recognize and support.

• **Why can't the protocol be simpler?**

It is possible that the protocol might be simplified. We are looking carefully at what is needed for best outcomes, and what is unnecessary. Many find that starting with a few basics and then adding other parts of the protocol over several months is an easy way to optimize. In addition, we recognize that many people do not like taking pills, so we have reduced the number of pills and capsules taken by combining most of the contents in a smoothie-type format. However, without successful intervention, Alzheimer's disease is a terminal illness, so unsurprisingly, when we were developing the initial treatment in 2011, we were desperate to find anything that might turn the tide. Therefore, we started by targeting all of the contributors—the "thirty-six holes in the roof"—but as we understand better which priorities are higher and which are lower for each person, we may be able to simplify the protocol. However, we must be cautious, since the price of failure is the loss of the patient. Therefore, for best outcomes, we continue to target as many of the identified contributors to cognitive decline as possible for each person.

For those who are interested in prevention—those who are asymptomatic and show no decline on cognitive testing—we have indeed developed a simpler protocol called PreCODE (for prevention of cognitive decline), since it is less complicated to prevent decline than to reverse it. This offers an incentive for all of us to begin a preventive protocol early, before cognitive symptoms occur. We recommend that everyone who is 45 years of age or older undergo a simple cognoscopy (specific blood tests, online cognitive testing, and an MRI, which is optional for those who are asymptomatic) and begin prevention.

- **How can you reduce the global burden of dementia in the most cost-effective way?**

The idea is to use a graduated approach. First, have as many people as possible on simple preventive measures (we developed PreCODE to provide the best results for prevention). Then the minority who develop cognitive decline despite prevention should begin a reversal program as early as possible (it is noteworthy that we have not documented a single case of dementia in those on prevention). The few who fail *that* undergo more extensive testing in order to begin a more extensive reversal program, with additional consultants to determine why there was failure in the initial reversal program. Finally, those rare individuals who fail even the more extensive program become inpatients in order to offer the most intensive evaluation and treatment. Thus the vast majority of people can be treated successfully inexpensively, and those who need more extensive evaluation and treatment will be identified. This graduated approach should minimize the overall cost to reduce the prevalence of dementia in any given population.

In addition to the questions, a number of people have leveled criticisms. As noted above, Aristotle said, "The only way to avoid criticism is to do nothing, say nothing, and be nothing." For those who read the book describing our initial protocol, *The End of Alzheimer's*, or the updated protocol in *The End of Alzheimer's Program*, 90 percent of the comments have been positive, 5 percent neutral, and 5 percent negative. Below are some of the criticisms:

* To suggest you can reverse cognitive decline is akin to telling a paraplegic that if he'd only follow a certain regime, he would grow his missing limb back.

Of course, paraplegic patients are not missing any limbs, they are simply paralyzed in their lower limbs. Setting aside that misunderstanding, many people expressed the belief that it is impossible to reverse cognitive decline. Indeed, this has been the standard line of the experts for many years. This is why we have been careful to document objective improvements and publish these in peer-reviewed journals. Thus we are not simply suggesting it, we have documented reversal of cognitive decline, published our findings about it, and most important, shown that the improvement is sustained. Furthermore, we have recently completed a clinical trial of the protocol, which provides further evidence for efficacy.

However, it is important to distinguish between results and expectations. We have never claimed that every single person gets better, and there are features that typically contribute to improvement as opposed to decline, such as compliance, the presence of toxins, and the degree of decline at presentation. So even though we have shown better results than have been achieved by any therapeutics previously, some people have been disappointed because they or their loved ones did not show improvement. I look forward to the day when every person does indeed show improvement. Meanwhile, we are continuing to research what are the critical variables that determine success or failure.

- **Although there are theoretical reasons why it might work, there is no empirical evidence for this approach.**

This is incorrect. As we noted immediately above, we have been careful to document our results and publish them in peer-reviewed journals. The background research appeared in over 220 published papers over the last four decades, and the clinical results were published in 2014, 2015, 2016, and 2018. These are all public-access papers, so they are freely available to all. Furthermore, some of the case studies were described in *The End of Alzheimer's*. I recommend that anyone who would like to see the empirical evidence simply read the published papers.

- **Conditions like leaky gut syndrome are treated as established fact, even though there is no evidence to support them.**

The National Library of Medicine of the United States lists 310 publications on leaky gut, journal articles going all the way back to 1984, so there is actually a mountain of evidence to support it. Not only is this a relatively well-established condition, it is one that plays an important role in producing systemic inflammation, and therefore there is increasing evidence that this condition plays a role in inflammatory bowel disease, cognitive decline, lupus, arthritis, and many other diseases. If after reading the 310 publications on leaky gut, you still do not believe this condition exists, then it may be of interest to talk with one of the experts in the field, such as Professor Alessio Fasano of Harvard University.

- **You cannot reverse Alzheimer's. At present the best all of the clinical trials hope for is being able to stop the cognitive decline in its tracks.**

Actually, the clinical trials of various drugs don't even attempt to stop the decline, which has been considered inevitable. They simply attempt to *slow* the decline, and in virtually every case, even that has failed (as noted in the introduction). The fundamental difference between these failed studies and the approach we developed is that the failed clinical trials attempted to treat Alzheimer's disease without addressing the actual contributors to it. This is like a mechanic attempting to fix every car that comes into the shop by filling it with high-octane gas, without determining what is actually wrong with the car. A few cars may run better for a time, but, no surprise, most will not, and the problems that brought the cars to the shop will not have been fixed.

* **Any effective interventions for common diseases would already be widely used.**

Doctors throughout the ages—from Semmelweis (who pioneered antiseptic procedures) to Paracelsus (the father of toxicology) to Lind (who found that citrus cures scurvy)—have proven this claim wrong. Therefore, this assumption—that any effective treatment for cognitive decline (or other common diseases) would immediately be in widespread use—ignores medical history and is exceedingly naive. As one of thousands of counterexamples, my wife and I witnessed this when our daughter developed lupus. We took her to two of the recognized experts, neither of whom had anything to offer except to watch her and determine when steroids should be started. There was simply no attempt to determine *why* she was developing lupus (are you starting to see a pattern here?). Desperate, we then took her to an integrative physician—one who was not famous the way the two experts were, not an acknowledged expert in lupus, not an authoritative academician—who readily determined *why* our daughter was developing lupus, and targeted the root cause. Our daughter has been free of lupus for a decade now. There are many, many examples like this, not only in lupus but in many other diseases such as rheumatoid arthritis, heart disease, type 2 diabetes, leaky gut (which, as noted above, some deny even exists despite hundreds of publications about it!), and yes, now in Alzheimer's.

Beyond interventions for common diseases, this sort of reasoning implies that our doctors always take whatever time is needed to evaluate and prescribe the best treatments for us, that our healthcare system always charges us only what is reasonable and appropriate, that our insurance companies always pay what they should, that the food we purchase at the grocery store is always healthy, that the medical system is not broken, that the thousands of toxins we are exposed to daily are nonexistent, and on and on . . . I look forward to the day that these naive beliefs reflect reality, but until then, the idea that the results we have published to date cannot be true simply because not all doctors are practicing our protocol (which, by the way, is in practice by over a thousand doctors already) is downright silly.

- **It would be an uphill battle to change our current medical system and pharmaceutical abuse.**

Sadly, this is true. But fundamental change is especially important for the very diseases without effective standard treatment—from autism to ALS to Alzheimer's. Twenty-first-century medicine is indeed changing the system, and with it, achieving results that have not been seen before. Let's keep the momentum and change the system for the better.

CHAPTER 9

Misconceptions and Misperceptions: Digging In Our Heals

By three methods we may learn wisdom:
first, by reflection, which is noblest;
second, by imitation, which is easiest;
and third by experience, which is the bitterest.

—CONFUCIUS

If there isn't thick-cut bacon in Heaven, why be good?

—ANONYMOUS

G rowing up in Florida, I was in the Greenback Surf Club—
an absolutely great group of teens like Bug, Hobby, and
Bermuda Schwartz. Since the surf in southern Florida is
generally poor, we would save our money from various odd jobs
such as lawn mower, parking valet, busboy, and encyclopedia
salesman so that we could surf spots in Puerto Rico, Hawaii, and
California. Meanwhile, on weekends we'd drive up the Florida
coast for the better surf in Cocoa Beach and Fort Pierce, rising at
three A.M. so we could surf at daybreak, when the waves were glass-
iest and often best.

As you can imagine, it was frequently difficult to stay alert driving home in the evening after getting up so early. On one trip, I was driving through Fort Pierce on the way home, with the other guys sleeping in the car. I came to a railroad crossing, and the crossbar was up, with no lights flashing or sounds, so being sleep deprived, I crossed as I looked down the track, instead of *after* looking down the track. Bad idea. As I looked up, I was shocked into alertness by seeing the train bearing down on us, about thirty feet from our car. Not particularly fast, but with plenty of speed to have killed us, of course . . . and as the car cleared the tracks and the train plowed into our backdraft, the crossbar came down, the red lights flashed, and the "ding-ding!" of the warning finally sounded. Earlier warning would have been appreciated.

It is of little value, of course, to activate the warning lights and the crossbar while the train is bisecting your car and sending its occupants to their afterlives. To make matters worse, the very presence of the open gate crossbar offers a false sense of security. And so it is with Alzheimer's—the Dementia Train is bearing down on us for decades, but we don't bother to look or respond until it is upon us. The drugs offer a false sense of security—a treatment we can prescribe—but in point of fact, those who take the drugs do *worse*, surprisingly, on the whole, than those who do not.

Because the fundamental nature of Alzheimer's disease and the many drivers of the process have not been understood, there have been many fallacious inferences, misguided recommendations, and naive assumptions. These have had a damaging impact on what research is funded, which drugs are developed, which clinical trials are approved, and how patients are treated—indeed, the entire belief system surrounding Alzheimer's disease. This is causing widespread harm to patients, unfortunately. As I mentioned in the introduction, the entire approach is backward.

This confusion is somewhat reminiscent of the ancient idea that the Earth is at the center of the universe. Of course this seemed reasonable to Earth dwellers, but it left paradoxes, like some of the planets seemed to move backward at times. Something was wrong, and the Greek astronomer Aristarchus of Samos suggested that perhaps the Earth actually revolved around the Sun— something considered crazy by many 2,300 years ago. Today we have paradox after paradox in Alzheimer's, again because the standard model is incompatible with the data.

Here are just a few of the misconceptions and misassumptions:

- **The cause of Alzheimer's disease is unknown.**

This is incorrect on two fronts. First, it assumes that there is a single cause of Alzheimer's, when the epidemiological research, the pathological research, and the microbiological research all argue that there is no single cause. Quite the opposite—there are many contributors, most of which are indeed known. It has been suggested that there may be an infectious cause of Alzheimer's, for example, but there has not even been agreement on which organism: is it *Herpes simplex*, HHV-6A (another *Herpes* virus), *Porphyromonas gingivalis* (from the periodontitis associated with poor dentition), *Borrelia* (the Lyme disease organism) or a related spirochete, a yeast such as *Candida*, various molds, or another pathogen? Nothing suggests that only one of these is "the cause" of Alzheimer's, whereas everything suggests they all may contribute to risk.

Beyond pathogens, however, there are many other contributors: insulin resistance, mercury and other toxins, vascular disease, trauma, reduced hormonal support, reduced nutrient support, reduced growth factor support, and on and on. Thus there is no evidence to support the notion that Alzheimer's disease has a single cause, and there is a great deal to support the notion that multiple known contributors play critical roles.

- **Alzheimer's disease is caused by amyloid. / Alzheimer's disease is caused by tau. / Alzheimer's disease is caused by misfolded proteins.**

In the 95 percent of cases in which Alzheimer's is sporadic (as opposed to the 5 percent in which it is familial—i.e., inherited), the amyloid that collects in the brains, the tau, and the misfolded proteins are all mediators, not causes. Sure, they are involved in the pathophysiology, but it is critical to recognize that these do not *start* the process. The process is started by the very pathogens and other contributors noted immediately above, and the amyloid is actually a protective response to these insults. This is a critical distinction, since removing the *cause* of Alzheimer's makes sense, whereas removing the *mediators* without first addressing the upstream cause(s) is at best a short-term solution. Indeed, removing the amyloid pharmacologically has proven to be a billion-dollar mistake.

- **The best way to treat Alzheimer's disease is with a drug.**

Neither theory nor practice supports this common misunderstanding. The pathophysiology of Alzheimer's disease is too complicated for a single drug to be the optimal treatment. Furthermore, the drugs used for Alzheimer's disease do not affect the actual contributors to the disease. The greatest promise for drug therapy is as part of an overall personalized, precision medicine protocol.

- **Because there is no effective prevention or treatment for Alzheimer's disease, there is no reason to check your ApoE status.**

This is a common misconception. Indeed, many clinicians recommend against this testing: "Most experts don't recommend genetic testing for late-onset Alzheimer's." Again, this is completely backward—you should not be waiting until you develop Alzheimer's to get genetic testing! Just as most people know their blood pressure and cholesterol—in order to minimize their risk for heart attacks and strokes—and most know their colonoscopy results— to prevent colon cancer—we should all know our ApoE status (0, 1, or 2 copies of ApoE4—that's what you want to know) so that we can minimize our risk for Alzheimer's. You may wish to check the website ApoE4.Info and correspond with some of the over 3,000 members with ApoE4, since the optimal technique for avoiding Alzheimer's is slightly different for those who are ApoE4-positive as opposed to those who are ApoE4-negative.

- **There is nothing that will prevent Alzheimer's disease.**

This is horribly out-of-date, yet is still being parroted by many, despite proof to the contrary—for example, from the FINGER study from Finland. There are actually many factors reducing risk, from plant-rich ketogenic diets to exercise to brain training to omega-3 unsaturated fats and many more. Furthermore, even though studies of generic prevention have yielded some good results, a superior approach is to identify the personal risk factors for each of us so that the prevention program can target the critical factors and ignore the other ones that are unimportant for each of us. For example, some of us have our major risk due to systemic inflammation, and therefore combining SPMs (specialized pro-resolving mediators) with removal of the inflammatory factor is a key part of the prevention program. Others of us have no significant systemic inflammation but have metabolic syndrome, which is readily addressable. Each of us thus has a different set of risk factors, and targeting these specifically is the rational way to go. We developed the PreCODE program for this optimal, personalized prevention.

- **There is no effective treatment for Alzheimer's disease.**

Again, this ubiquitous statement shows how archaic the current standard of care is. Because the underlying pathophysiology of Alzheimer's disease is ongoing for twenty years before a diagnosis, the last thing we want to do is to sit and watch for those twenty years as the person advances through the presymptomatic stage (at which we can easily pick up risk factors and prevent decline) to the SCI stage (subjective cognitive impairment, which often lasts a decade and is reversible virtually 100 percent of the time) to the MCI stage (which often lasts several years and is usually reversible) to finally reach a diagnosis of Alzheimer's disease (which can still be improved in some cases, but there is no reason to wait that long, and every reason to intervene earlier). By definition, a person does not have Alzheimer's disease until he or she begins to lose his/her ability to perform activities of daily living, such as bathing. Therefore, it is barbaric to wait for anyone to reach the stage at which a diagnosis of Alzheimer's disease is made. This is like watching someone's tumor advance until it is widely metastatic. Alzheimer's disease should be a very rare condition, and the fact that many clinicians are telling patients that nothing can be done is causing patients to delay seeking treatment, affecting outcomes negatively.

Furthermore, we have repeatedly published well-documented examples of the reversal of cognitive decline, so at some point, ignoring a peer-reviewed, published, effective treatment in favor of a proven-ineffective treatment begins to look like negligence.

- **When we evaluate patients with cognitive decline, we seek to determine whether the correct diagnosis is Alzheimer's disease or a treatable cause of dementia, such as vitamin B_{12} deficiency.**

The assumption that various contributors such as vitamin B_{12} deficiency, vitamin D deficiency, estradiol deficiency, and dozens of others are completely independent from Alzheimer's disease is simplistic. Sure, there is a different pathology for pure vitamin B_{12} deficiency, but in the vast majority of cases, it is not pure, but is associated with an increase in homocysteine, which in turn is associated with an increased risk for Alzheimer's disease. Many such factors may serve as contributors, as I've noted before, from infections to toxins to reductions in growth factors, hormones, nutrients, oxygenation, and blood flow. Furthermore, recognizing these contributors reveals that Alzheimer's disease *is* a treatable cause of dementia, especially when treated "early"—which means during the first ten to fifteen years of pathophysiology, so the therapeutic window is quite large.

- **We check thyroid and B12 on patients with cognitive decline. Since Alzheimer's is untreatable, there is no need for detailed testing.**

Unfortunately, this is a common practice. How can you treat a disease without knowing what is causing it? Twenty-first-century medicine is precision medicine, in which the mechanisms of any given cancer or neurodegenerative disease or other illness are first identified and then targeted. So if you are being evaluated for cognitive decline, or risk for decline, and your practitioner is not assessing your hs-CRP, HOMA-IR, free T3 and reverse T3, vitamin D, heavy metals, organic toxins, biotoxins, CIRS markers, and vascular markers such as LDL particle number or triglyceride-to-HDL ratio, then you may wish to talk to him or her about more extensive testing to determine what is causing the decline or risk for decline.

- **If you plan to use a treatment protocol for patients, then each intervention alone must have been proven to exert a significant effect.**

This is the current standard, and it is based on faulty reasoning, which assumes that the brain is a linear system—in other words, you can take each single pill or treatment and analyze it separately, then simply add up the effects. By the same rationale, if you don't see much effect from any single treatment, then a combination of, say, ten or twenty of those ingredients that didn't show much alone cannot have any effect. The brain is much more complicated than that! This is like saying that to get to your friend's house, you need to go out of your driveway and take a left, then a right, then a right, then a left. To test this, you go out of your driveway and take a left, then look to see if you can see your friend's house; then you come out of your driveway again and take a right, and see if you can see it; then you come out of your driveway yet again and take a right and see if you can see the house; then one last time with that final left. Doing each of these turns by itself is not the same as putting them all together! And the same is true for a treatment protocol—you can't simply add up the effects of each single intervention! Putting it all together in a coordinated fashion is the key.

These are just a few of the many misunderstandings—misunderstandings that impact evaluation, treatment, prevention, and the entire philosophy surrounding Alzheimer's disease.

So please, let's quit saying that there is nothing that can prevent, delay, or reverse cognitive decline in Alzheimer's disease. And let's quit saying that there is no reason to have your ApoE genetics evaluated. And let's quit saying that Alzheimer's is "caused by misfolded proteins." And let's quit saying that a single drug cure for Alzheimer's is just around the corner. And let's quit saying that a drug that barely slows decline and improves no one is "what we've been searching for." Let's reconsider the way we think about Alzheimer's disease.

CHAPTER 10

Quantified Self and the Reversal of Cognitive Decline

Vision without execution is hallucination.

—THOMAS EDISON

The twenty-first century is the Century of Biology, and we are now in the Era of the Quantified Self. Just as engineering has allowed us to search the internet and hold Zoom meetings, biomedicine is increasingly allowing us to determine our health status and risks, often simply, longitudinally, and actionably. Used optimally, typically with the aid of a medical practitioner or health coach (although this is not absolutely necessary—there is a remarkable amount you can do yourself), this information can save your brain and keep you sharp for decades. Some of the many examples of what we can all assess include:

- Blood pressure and pulse (e.g., Omron blood pressure monitor)
- Body temperature continuous monitoring (e.g., Oura ring)

- Body fat (e.g., skinfold calipers or bioimpedance)
- Movement and exercise tracking (e.g., Apple Watch or Fitbit)
- Oxygen saturation, nocturnal and diurnal (e.g., Apple Watch or Beddr)
- Heart rate variability (e.g., Apple Watch)
- Vascular elasticity (e.g., iHeart)
- EKG (e.g., Apple Watch)
- Sleep time and stages (e.g., Oura ring)
- Serum glucose (e.g., Precision Xtra)
- Continuous glucose monitoring (e.g., FreeStyle Libre, with prescription)
- Ketones (beta-hydroxybutyrate in serum, acetone on breath, or acetoacetate in urine—e.g., Biosense breathalyzer for breath acetone)
- Nutritional analysis (macro and micro—e.g., Cronometer)
- Toxin presence in cosmetics and personal products (e.g., Think Dirty app)
- Online cognitive assessments and processing speed (e.g., CNS Vital Signs)
- Speech changes associated with various disease states (e.g., Canary Speech or Vocalis)
- Genomics, with analysis for many risk factors and personal characteristics (e.g., 23andMe, with analysis by Promethease or IntellxxDNA or Genetic Genie)
- Telomere length (e.g., TA-65 or Life Length)
- Gut microbiome (e.g., Viome)
- Oral microbiome (e.g., OralDNA)
- Colorectal cancer screen (e.g., Cologuard)

The ability we all now have to measure these various parameters—and more are on the way, no doubt—is actually a lifesaver, and here's why: unlike in the twentieth century, when many people died of acute illnesses such as pneumonia, virtually all of us are now dying of chronic illnesses such as cardiovascular disease, cancer, or Alzheimer's. The bad news is that these diseases often do not produce symptoms until they are so far advanced that they are difficult to treat. As I mentioned earlier, Alzheimer's disease is typically diagnosed about twenty years after the brain changes begin, so that what we used to think of as a disease of our 60s, 70s, and 80s is actually a disease of our 40s, 50s, and 60s, whose diagnosis is unfortunately delayed for twenty years. The worse news is that most of our doctors are not checking these vital parameters, so we are being allowed to progress to the late, symptomatic stages of chronic illnesses before any action is taken. Literally we are being allowed to die silently over the decades.

The good news about chronic illnesses is that we can see them coming for years ahead of time, if we just bother to look. That's where these various health parameters really shine. We can all follow our status, pick up early decline at a time when it's simple to make a major difference, and track our own progress as we improve. And here's an exciting dividend—tracking and tweaking over the years improves our performance, health, appearance, and longevity. What's not to like?

Just as with triangulation, obtaining multiple data points is powerful, and combining genomic data (for example, are you ApoE4-positive? Do you have effective or ineffective detox genetics? Do you have a propensity for blood clotting?), biochemical data (for example, do you have ongoing inflammation? Is your lipid profile abnormal? Do you have prediabetes?), and longitudinal quantified-self data (which now can be included in an app) delivers a potent combination, allowing a much clearer look at what is driving cognitive change or risk for change. These data can help your health coach, practitioner, and you to chart the best course for your cognition for years to come.

There are now over 5,000 people who have adopted the ReCODE Protocol, and their responses have helped us to continue to enhance the approach. One of the lessons learned is that it is important to determine which parameters are highest priority and which are much lower priority. Practitioners and patients sometimes focus on lower priority goals and thus miss the critical parameters necessary for success. Although this varies from person to person, and therefore is dependent on each person's evaluation, there are key considerations for all, and I've listed these in order of priority below:

1. Energetics

As I mentioned in the introduction, the essence of Alzheimer's disease is a chronic or repeated insufficiency—there is not enough support for a network that is critical for neuroplasticity. PET scans from patients with Alzheimer's show reduced glucose metabolism in a characteristic pattern in the temporal lobe (inside your temple region) and parietal lobe (running up behind your ears), and in fact this pattern may appear a decade or even more before the diagnosis of Alzheimer's disease.

Bridging this energy gap—the gap between supply and demand—is critical for improving cognition. As Dr. Stephen Cunnane has shown, ketones provide an alternative energy source to the usual glucose—which is critical because the vast majority of patients with Alzheimer's have insulin resistance and therefore do not utilize glucose normally—and thus can bridge the energy gap, which is why ketosis is such an important part of our overall protocol. The target level is 1.0–4.0 mM BHB (beta-hydroxybutyrate), which you can measure with a finger stick and ketone meter, or you can use an accurate breathalyzer such as Biosense, in which case the target is over 7 ACES, and over 10 ACES at least once per day (all laboratory targets are listed on pages 21–24 of *The End of Alzheimer's Program*).

Since this energy deficit has typically been ongoing for years before symptoms of cognitive decline, it is paramount to bridge this gap as quickly as possible, and therefore, starting by taking ketones is the best way to go in the short run, whereas in the long run, we want to produce our own ketones, which is what happens when we use our own fat for energy.

So you need energy, and to get that you need to deliver the fuel and then burn it to give you the energy. What this means is that you need not only the ketones, but also good blood flow to your brain (cerebral blood flow), good oxygen saturation (target 96% or higher), and good mitochondrial function (function of your cells' "batteries," which turn your fuel into energy).

For cerebral blood flow, you can check your vascular risk factors: it is best to have a triglyceride-to-HDL ratio <1.3:1, so, for example, if your HDL is 60 mg/dL, your triglycerides should be <78 mg/dL. If you check LDL-P (LDL particle number), it should be in the 700–1200 nM range. Your cerebral blood flow can be increased with exercise, with EWOT (exercise with oxygen therapy), and by improving vascular compromise by resolving inflammation and hitting the lipid targets just mentioned. In addition, vascular dilation can be enhanced with nitric oxide, which you can increase with exercise, beetroot juice, arginine, or Neo40, as well as other vasodilators such as ginkgo or vinpocetine. For those with a tendency for increased blood clotting, nattokinase and pycnogenol can be used.

For oxygen saturation, one of the most common contributors to cognitive decline is unrecognized oxygen desaturation, which is usually at night. This is not just for those with sleep apnea, although that is a common contributor. While we are sleeping—targeting eight hours of sleep (and you can check your sleep timing and even sleep stages on the Oura ring; you can also check your sleep timing on the Apple Watch)—our oxygen saturation should be 96–98 percent. As your average oxygen saturation drops at night, there is a direct correlation with brain shrinkage in specific areas, including the hippocampus, which is critical for memory formation and heavily impacted in Alzheimer's. You can check your oxygen saturation on an Apple Watch or on an oximeter like that from Beddr, or on an oximeter from your physician, or you can have this checked during a sleep study.

For mitochondrial function, there is no simple test, although you can get a general idea by testing organic acids. Mitochondrial support includes increasing your NAD (nicotinamide adenine dinucleotide) with nicotinamide riboside—this provides energy for your mitochondria; increasing your number of mitochondria with PQQ (pyrroloquinoline quinone); and increasing a critical factor in mitochondrial function, called ubiquinol. In addition, there is intriguing work suggesting that you can boost your mitochondrial function by taking methylene blue, and this may prove to be an important addition to the treatment of cognitive decline.

It is difficult to overstate the importance of energetics for those of us with cognitive decline or risk for decline. Practitioners and brain health coaches can help to achieve the best outcomes.

2. Insulin sensitivity

When we grow brain cells in petri dishes in the lab, we always include insulin because it is a potent survival factor for the neurons. Therefore, it is no surprise that when your brain cells become unresponsive or poorly responsive to insulin, your neurons do not survive as well. In fact, the molecules carrying the insulin signal in your brain actually undergo a measurable physical change (due to phosphorylation of serine and threonine on IRS-1) when you develop insulin resistance. Professor Ed Goetzl has shown that virtually all people with Alzheimer's disease are insulin resistant in their brains, whether or not they are insulin resistant peripherally. Such resistance is a key contributor to cognitive decline, but fortunately we have a large arsenal to combat insulin resistance and return us to insulin sensitivity.

Testing for insulin resistance is straightforward—you simply want to know your fasting glucose and your fasting insulin, and that allows a simple calculation of HOMA-IR (which stands for homeostatic model assessment of insulin resistance), which is a measure of insulin resistance. Here's an example. Let's say your fasting glucose is 100 mg/dL and your fasting insulin is 10 mIU/L. You simply multiply these together and divide by 405 to get your HOMA-IR, so here it would be $(100)(10)/405 = 2.4$. This indicates insulin resistance—the target is <1.2. Let's now say you adopted the protocol and improved your glucose status. You now may have a fasting glucose of 80 and a fasting insulin of 5, which would give you an excellent HOMA-IR of just under 1.0, showing that you are now insulin sensitive. You can do this!

Becoming insulin sensitive is also straightforward, and it starts with the KetoFLEX 12/3 diet we have described, which is a plant-rich, high-fiber, mildly ketogenic diet that avoids grains, dairy, and simple carbohydrates and includes fasting of twelve to sixteen hours overnight and three hours before bedtime. When such a diet is combined with regular exercise (include some weight training, because muscle is rich in insulin receptors and thus increases your insulin sensitivity), the good sleep noted above, and stress reduction, this is typically enough to produce insulin sensitivity.

For those who remain insulin resistant, there are many additions that can be helpful. First, it's an excellent idea to see what may be spiking your glucose and what may be cratering it, since both high glucose and low glucose (as it drops into the 50s and below) can contribute to cognitive decline. This is done by CGM—continuous glucose monitoring—which your practitioner can order for you. This follows your glucose for a few weeks, so you can see how you respond to various foods, and whether you are becoming hypoglycemic at night (which is surprisingly common for those on standard American diets). Alternatively, you can check your own glucose easily with a drop of blood from a finger stick, using the Precision Xtra glucose meter or a similar device.

Support for insulin sensitivity can be enhanced with zinc, magnesium, chromium picolinate, Ceylon cinnamon, berberine, N-acetyl cysteine, metformin, bergamot oil, or bitter melon, among others. Your practitioner and health coach can help you optimize your insulin sensitivity. In rare cases, although insulin sensitivity will be achieved, the insulin levels may be too low to avoid prediabetes (typically this is with insulin levels down at 1–2 mIU/L). In those cases, your physician may consider increasing endogenous insulin with Victoza or Januvia.

Virtually all of us can become insulin sensitive, and this is a critical goal in the reversal of cognitive decline, since insulin resistance (which affects 80 million Americans) is one of the most common contributors to dementia.

3. Trophic support

In addition to energy and insulin sensitivity, your brain needs to receive supportive survival signals, and these come from three sources: growth factors like nerve growth factor (NGF) and brain-derived neurotrophic factor (BDNF); hormones like estrogen, testosterone, and thyroid hormone; and nutrients like vitamin B_{12}, vitamin D, and the omega-3 fat DHA (docosahexaenoic acid). The target for omega-3 fats is at least 10 percent (omega-3 index), and the ratio for inflammatory omega-6 fats to anti-inflammatory omega-3 fats is from 1:1 up to 4:1. If you are drifting up to 10:1 or 15:1 omega-6:omega-3, which is common with standard American diets, then you may be hurting yourself with too much inflammatory fat.

One easy way we can all use to follow our nutritional status is a website called Cronometer. This tracks not only macronutrients such as protein, carbohydrates, and fats, but also micronutrients such as vitamin D and choline. If you try this, you may find quickly what so many of us find—that we are not getting enough of key nutrients and minerals, such as choline, zinc, magnesium, iodine, omega-3 fats, and fiber. All of these turn out to play important roles in cognition: choline, for example, is required for the synthesis of the most important memory-related neurotransmitter, acetylcholine. We should be getting about 550 mg of choline per day, which we can obtain from foods like eggs, liver, meat, beans, and nuts; or from supplements like citicoline or alpha-GPC (alpha-glycerylphosphorylcholine).

You can check your hormone levels easily, as well as nutrient levels, and use these to optimize the various brain supports. However, there is no clinical test for brain levels of NGF and BDNF, although there is a serum test for BDNF. You can increase your NGF with ALCAR (acetyl-L-carnitine) or *Hericium erinaceus* (lion's mane mushroom), and increase your BDNF with exercise and/or whole coffee fruit extract (WCFE).

A recent addition to this list of brain-critical growth factors, hormones, and nutrients is another type of cognition-supporting fat, called plasmalogens. These are reduced in patients with Alzheimer's, and restoring normal levels holds promise as part of an effective protocol to prevent and reverse cognitive decline (as mentioned in Julie's story in chapter 7). Biochemist Dr. Dayan Goodenowe and the company Prodrome now offer evaluation for plasmalogen levels, as well as supplements to increase these levels. You can also increase your plasmalogen levels with some seafoods such as scallops.

Finally, you may wish to talk with your practitioner about peptides with trophic effects. There is remarkable potential for many of these, especially when delivered intranasally to enhance brain penetration. Some have only been tested as monotherapies, unfortunately, and therefore would not be expected to exert much effect without addressing other features of the neurodegenerative process. Some examples of these neurotrophic peptides include Cerebrolysin, Davunetide, and thymosin beta-4.

You can see how many different suboptimal factors may

contribute to the network insufficiency called Alzheimer's disease. Just as it takes the coordination of many different complementary departments to make a company run smoothly, it takes the coordination of many different systems and functions to sustain cognition. Supplying the necessary energy involves oxygenation, blood flow, ketones, and mitochondrial support; this must be coupled with insulin sensitivity and trophic support, as well as the other critical functions discussed immediately below.

4. Resolution of inflammation and prevention of further inflammation

The COVID-19 pandemic has reminded all of us how damaging inflammation can be, as so many deaths have been attributed to the cytokine storm associated with inflammation. The inflammation associated with Alzheimer's and pre-Alzheimer's (MCI and SCI) is of course much more chronic and includes the production of the amyloid itself. Therefore, as long as inflammation is ongoing, you are continuing to produce the Alzheimer's-associated amyloid and are at risk for continued cognitive decline. Conversely, resolving the inflammation is an effective ameliorative process as part of the overall protocol.

You can check your inflammation status by having a blood test for hs-CRP (high-sensitivity C-reactive protein, also referred to as cardiac CRP). It is best for your hs-CRP to be below 0.9 mg/dL. Additional, optional tests for inflammation include A/G ratio (albumin-to-globulin ratio: target 1.8 or higher), ESR (erythrocyte sedimentation rate), TNF-alpha (tumor necrosis factor alpha), IL-6 (interleukin 6), and ferritin (which is an iron storage protein, but also increases with inflammation), among others.

There are three steps to removing inflammation as a contributor to cognitive decline:

1. Resolving the ongoing inflammation
2. Removing the source(s) of the inflammation
3. Preventing new inflammation

You can resolve the ongoing inflammation with SPMs (specialized pro-resolving mediators), which are available over the counter. Alternatively, you can use high doses of omega-3 fats, such as 2 to 4 grams of omega-3 from fish oil or krill oil. Typically, taking the SPMs for one to two months is sufficient to resolve the inflammation.

It is critical, however, to identify the source of inflammation so that you can prevent recurrence. For some, this will be metabolic syndrome (which combines inflammation with increased cholesterol, LDL, and triglycerides; insulin resistance; increased waist circumference; and hypertension), for others, leaky gut or oral pathogens ("leaky gums" due to gingivitis or periodontitis) or chronic sinusitis or infections such as Lyme disease or another of the tick-borne organisms. These can all be identified with standard blood tests, stool testing, sinus cultures, and an OralDNA test for the oral microbiome. In addition, poor sleep is associated with inflammation, so as noted above, checking and optimizing sleep are important, as well.

Metabolic syndrome is reversible with a low-carbohydrate, anti-inflammatory diet, fasting (twelve to sixteen hours each night or one day each week) and exercise, best combined with gut healing (using bone broth or DGL—deglycyrrhizinated licorice—and ProButyrate). Leaky gut is usually treatable with a combination of gut healing and treatment of pathogens involved in dysbiosis, such as *Candida*. Oral pathogens can be treated with a combination of Dentalcidin toothpaste and mouthwash, oral probiotics (e.g., Revitin), and referral to an oral-systemic dental specialist. For specific organisms such as fungal sinusitis or tick-borne organisms, treating with targeted antimicrobials is key to removing the source of inflammation.

Anti-inflammatories are then helpful to prevent future inflammation. These may include omega-3 fats such as EPA (eicosapentaenoic acid), curcumin, ginger, alpha-lipoic acid, and anti-inflammatory diets, among others. LDN (low-dose naltrexone) also reduces inflammation and supports the immune system, as does the peptide thymosin alpha-1. We generally avoid aspirin and other COX inhibitors (cyclooxygenase inhibitors) because of their side effects of damage to the gut lining and kidneys.

5. Treatment of pathogens, optimization of microbiomes

As noted above, chronic inflammation associated with the cognitive decline of Alzheimer's disease may be caused by chronic infections. In fact, the beta-amyloid that collects in the brains of Alzheimer's patients has been shown to be an antimicrobial peptide, so as you are fighting these various infections, you are making the amyloid of Alzheimer's as part of your body's strategy to kill infectious agents. Therefore, identifying and targeting these various infections represents another important part of the optimal protocol for reversal of cognitive decline.

Some of the infectious agents that have been associated with Alzheimer's disease include, as I mentioned in the last chapter, *Herpes simplex* (from cold sores), *HHV-6A* (a *Herpes* virus that may enter through the sinuses) and other *Herpes* family viruses, *Porphyromonas gingivalis* (from poor dentition), *Borrelia* (from Lyme disease), other tick-borne infections (*Bartonella, Babesia, Ehrlichia*), other spirochetes such as *Treponema denticola* (another oral pathogen), and various fungi such as the yeast *Candida* and molds such as *Stachybotrys, Penicillium, Aspergillus,* and *Chaetomium.* Your practitioner can test for these by culturing or by antibody testing, and then initiate specific treatment focused on the pathogen identified.

Beyond the destruction of pathogens, it is important to support healthy microbiomes, using probiotics and prebiotics. Probiotics are available for the gut microbiome, the oral microbiome, and the sinus microbiome, and optimal microbiomes in turn exert multiple salutary effects, from inhibiting pathogens to producing vital metabolic products and strengthening physiological barriers. Prebiotics—the food that supports the microbiome—are available from foods (such as asparagus, onions, garlic, leeks, and dandelion greens) or as supplements (such as organic psyllium husk and the konjac root of PGX).

6. Detoxification

The most difficult area of expertise to master in the reversal of cognitive decline is detoxification, and the patients that have severe toxic exposure are the most difficult to treat successfully. However, with diligence, detail orientation, and continued tweaking, many do indeed improve, and sustain their improvement.

The toxins to which we are all exposed fall into three groups: (1) metals and other inorganics, like air pollutants; (2) organics, such as benzene, toluene, and glyphosate; (3) biotoxins, i.e., toxins produced by organisms, such as the mycotoxins produced by certain mold species. We are exposed to toxins and toxicants in our moldy homes and places of work, in the air pollution we breathe, in the pesticide- and herbicide-laden foods we eat, the beauty products we use, the impure water we drink, the printers and other electronic devices in our homes, and even in the receipts and other products we touch. Beyond this, there are potential "physical toxins" such as the ubiquitous Wi-Fi signals to which we are all exposed.

You can check your metal status using Quicksilver, which has a Tri-Test for mercury and an all-metals test for other metals such as lead, cadmium, iron, and copper, as well as the metalloid arsenic. Alternatively, you can get a test from Doctor's Data, Lab-Corp, or another group. For organic toxins, Great Plains Laboratory offers a urinary test, and for biotoxins, RealTime Labs and Great Plains both offer urinary mycotoxin tests. You can also test your home or workplace for the specific molds that produce mycotoxins, such as *Stachybotrys, Aspergillus, Penicillium, Chaetomium,* and *Wallemia,* by obtaining an ERMI score (Environmental Protection Agency Relative Moldiness Index; goal <2) or HERTSMI-2 score (Health Effects Roster of Type-Specific Formers of Mycotoxins and Inflammagens—2nd Version; goal <11). You can obtain these at mycometrics.com or via other mold testing groups.

Beyond direct tests for toxins, it's helpful to know how you are responding to any toxin exposure (and we all have some degree of toxin exposure, unfortunately) and whether your genes are good ones or not such good ones for detoxification. This is reflected in your immune activation, assessed by C4a, TGF-beta-1 (transforming growth factor beta-1), and MMP-9 (matrix metalloprotease-9); your detoxification status, assessed by glutathione level and tests of toxin effects on your liver, kidneys, and blood (such as ALT, AST, GGT, creatinine, BUN, platelet count, white blood cell count, and hematocrit); and your detoxification genetics (e.g., from IntellxxDNA or 23andMe with Promethease or Genetic Genie, for example).

For detoxification, there are basic guidelines we can all adopt:

- Filtered water, 1 to 4 liters each day.

- Sweating, whether from exercise or sauna (preferably infrared) or anything else, followed by showering with a nontoxic soap such as castile, an excellent way to reduce toxin load.

- Plant-rich high-fiber diet, with detoxifying vegetables such as broccoli, Brussels sprouts, cauliflower, kale, cabbage, lemon, ginger, garlic, artichoke, and beetroot.

- Detoxifying supplements such as sulforaphane, vitamin C, and guggul.

- Eat organic fruits and vegetables, especially for the Environmental Working Group's Dirty Dozen, which represents the greatest exposure to pesticides: strawberries, spinach, kale, nectarines, apples, grapes, peaches, cherries, pears, tomatoes, celery, and potatoes. In contrast, the EWG's Clean Fifteen are less of a concern for pesticide exposure because they have more protection than the Dirty Dozen and are therefore not as important to buy organic: avocados, sweet corn, pineapples, onions, papayas, frozen sweet peas, eggplant, asparagus, cauliflower, cantaloupes, broccoli, mushrooms, cabbage, honeydew melon, and kiwi.

• Avoid eating high-mercury fish; these are the ones with long lives and large mouths (and thus high on the food chain), such as tuna, shark, and swordfish. Focus instead on the SMASH fish: salmon, mackerel (but not king mackerel), anchovies, sardines, and herring.

• Avoid the ingestion of dementogens in food, such as pesticides and herbicides (including glyphosate) from nonorganic fruits and vegetables, acrylamide in chips and fries, heat-treated arsenic in some chicken and some rice, antibiotics and hormones in some meats, bisphenol A (BPA) in canned foods, trans fats in many fried and baked foods, nitrites and nitrates in hot dogs and other processed meats, sulfates in processed foods, preservatives, and dyes, as well as sugar, high-fructose corn syrup, and other simple carbohydrates.

• Avoid cooking processes that produce toxic by-products, such as blackening meat, use of heat-treated oils, and use of trans fat oils.

• Avoid dental amalgams, which have a high mercury content.

- Use a HEPA filter such as IQAir, filtering both particulates and gases. For those of us who have been exposed to the California fires or to other forms of air pollution, it's especially important to have the HEPA filters operating when the air quality is poor.

- Avoid smoking and secondhand smoke.

- Avoid general anesthesia to the greatest extent possible, and prepare for general anesthesia by optimizing glutathione and overall detox.

- Focus on diaphragmatic breathing (from your belly rather than the intercostal muscles of your chest), and inhale through your nose rather than through your mouth.

- Avoid toxins in health and beauty aids. The app Think Dirty will give you an idea of what toxins are in each product. You may also wish to consult the Environmental Working Group database for its recommendations.

- Avoid toxins such as phthalates, dioxins, vinyl chloride, and BPA in plastics, and instead use storage vessels made of materials such as glass. Note that receipt paper is also a source of BPA.

- Avoid the lead from some paints and old plumbing.

- Manage and resolve stress, since toxin-related cognitive decline is associated with hypersensitivity to stress, often leading to setbacks in cognition.

- Massage may be useful to improve lymphatic flow and support detox.

- Support your detoxifying organs—liver and kidneys. For the liver, milk thistle is helpful, and some people also include curcumin, TUDCA (tauroursodeoxycholic acid), organic apples (which contain pectin, a toxin-binding agent), walnuts, avocados, pastured eggs, sardines, cruciferous vegetables, salad greens, artichokes, and fish oil. For the kidneys, beetroot juice, ginkgo, blueberries, gotu kola, and magnesium citrate are all helpful.

In addition to these general practices, target specific identified toxins such as trichothecenes (from the mold *Stachybotrys*) or organic mercury (from seafood) or benzene. For biotoxins, there are excellent books by Dr. Ritchie Shoemaker and Dr. Neil Nathan. For chemotoxins, Dr. Joseph Pizzorno has written a superb manual, *The Toxin Solution*.

I realize that it sounds as if toxins are everywhere and unavoidable, but please remember that this is a dynamic situation. We are all exposed constantly, but also detoxifying constantly, so the goal here is simply to reduce the toxin exposure enough and increase your detox capability enough that you are on the right side of the balance, rather than continually increasing your overall toxic burden. Reducing this burden will reduce your risk for cognitive decline, cancer, diabetes, and other chronic illnesses.

7. Stimulation

Just as working out improves physical health, brain stimulation of one form or another is often associated with best outcomes for those with cognitive decline. There are several different methods of stimulation, all of which have shown benefit. Brain training, such as that offered by BrainHQ (and its many programs, such as Hawk Eye and Double Decision) or Elevate, represents one form of brain stimulation. For best results, avoid major stress during brain training—if it's not possible to do 30 minutes three or four times per week without a lot of stress, then you can work up to this slowly. Light stimulation, such as that provided by Vielight (the gamma version was designed for those with cognitive decline) or by laser stimulation, represents another form. Magnetic stimulation, such as MeRT, represents a third method of brain stimulation. Sound stimulation (which appears to be best at 40 hertz) is a fourth method.

8. Immune support

In both COVID-19 and Alzheimer's, a high degree of inflammation coupled with a poor adaptive immune response is associated with a poor outcome. Therefore, we want to remove any identified inflammagens such as the pathogens described in point 5 above and any biotoxins noted in point 6 above, minimize inflammation, and provide support for the adaptive immune system. This includes optimizing vitamins A, C, and D (with K2) levels, zinc, quercetin,

N-acetyl cysteine, glutathione, R-lipoic acid, and beta-glucan. In addition, avoid the very lifestyle features that harm your immunity, including chronic stress (periods of acute stress with resolution are not nearly as harmful as chronic stress) and poor sleep.

9. Reducing beta-amyloid

The beta-amyloid that has been vilified in Alzheimer's disease, and removed with the antibodies (such as solanezumab, crenezumab, and aducanumab) without improving patients, is an antimicrobial, protective response. Therefore, removing the amyloid without first removing the various insults is potentially dangerous, and indeed we have seen several patients who declined in temporal association with antibody administration.

However, as noted earlier, the idea of reducing amyloid *after* removing the various identified insults is appealing, and this is where the anti-amyloid drugs may turn out to be very valuable (although none is yet approved, pending the FDA decision on aducanumab, due by June 2021). In addition, there are other agents that are useful for reducing the amyloid burden, such as curcumin, cat's claw, ashwagandha, resveratrol, and omega-3 fats.

10. Synaptogenesis and regeneration

After the various contributors to cognitive decline listed above have been addressed, it must be remembered that most people with cognitive decline have suffered the loss of millions of synaptic connections before even seeking help. Therefore, supporting the remaining synapses, enhancing function for those that are present but nonfunctional, and potentially restoring lost synapses are all crucial goals.

Part of this support is described in point 3 above, providing trophic support through growth factors (such as BDNF and NGF), hormones, and nutrients. In addition, stem cells may help with regeneration, and trials of stem cells for patients with Alzheimer's disease are ongoing. However, administering stem cells without addressing the ongoing causes of Alzheimer's is like trying to re-build a house as it's burning down—you are likely to have better results if you first put out the fire and then begin the rebuilding. Therefore, even if the ongoing trials fail, it may be productive to determine whether stem cells are effective after removing the various contributors to cognitive decline.

There are three types of stem cell approaches: embryonic stem cells, mesenchymal stem cells, and induced pluripotent stem cells (iPSC). All three of these show promise in the long run, although the iPSC face safety hurdles such as proving that they do not represent risk for tumor formation. Meanwhile, ongoing clinical trials are listed at ClinicalTrials.gov.

SUMMARY

Prevention and reversal of cognitive decline are now ongoing for many hundreds of people, just as they are for the seven survivors in this book. We now understand what the causes of cognitive decline are, so we can identify them and address them successfully. This is not easy—indeed, just as for any complicated machine or country or organ, there are many coordinated systems that must be intact and working for effective function—but it is feasible for virtually anyone with an experienced practitioner, a cognitive health coach (which in some cases may be one's spouse or relative or friend), and determination.

We have an unprecedented ability to follow our own key physiological parameters in order to optimize our brain health—our blood pressure, oxygen saturation, sleep quantity and quality, pulse and heart rate variability, EKG, nutrient intake, body mass index, fasting glucose, ketone level, caloric expenditure, genomics, cognitive assessment, and microbiomes, among other parameters. This helps us to optimize our nervous system function and prevent decline, and also lets us know in plenty of time if we need to consult a physician, instead of waiting until the neurodegenerative process has been ongoing for decades. This combination renders dementia optional instead of ineluctable and can truly help to make Alzheimer's a rare disease, as it should be.

All of the critical mechanisms underlying cognitive decline can be assessed and addressed:

- Energetics
- Insulin sensitivity
- Trophic support
- Inflammation
- Pathogens
- Toxins
- Brain stimulation
- Immune support

- Beta-amyloid
- Regeneration

Most important, you do not need to do everything perfectly for an excellent outcome. Simply get over the threshold to begin to see cognitive improvements. You can then continue to improve with ongoing optimization over time.

CHAPTER 11

Adaptation, Application:
Might Other Diseases Respond?

You are not expected to complete your life's work during your lifetime; neither are you excused from it.

—RABBI TARFON

Do I push the envelope? I break the envelope.

—GARRY MCFADDEN, *I AM HOMICIDE*

When I was completing my neurological training, a famous Nobel laureate came to visit our university, looking for a newly minted neurologist for a project he had in mind. His wife had been diagnosed with a rare neurodegenerative condition, and he wanted to hire someone to search the world over for outside-the-box treatments that might be of help to her. I was touched by his caring for his wife, and when I met with him, he pointed out that very few therapeutic attempts had ever been made on someone with her condition, so how did anyone know if something relatively straightforward might have been missed? He made a good point. Perhaps we have all been missing a basic pattern or concept or therapeutic approach that could allow us to treat the various neurodegenerative diseases successfully. Our research suggested that this might just possibly be the case.

One of the most common questions I am asked is whether the ReCODE approach we developed for cognitive decline is effective for other neurodegenerative diseases such as Parkinson's disease, Lewy body dementia, and ALS (amyotrophic lateral sclerosis, which is also called Lou Gehrig's disease). While we do not yet have enough data to know the answer to that question, a pattern is nonetheless emerging, one that I hope is pointing us in the right direction for prevention and reversal of decline in each of the neurodegenerative diseases.

First, it is important to distinguish between diseases for which there is effective treatment—such as some forms of cancer—and those for which there is no effective treatment. Neurodegenerative diseases fall into the latter category, and indeed, these represent the area of greatest biomedical failure when it comes to therapeutics. This means that the current standard of care is unhelpful, and thus adhering to the standard of care guarantees failure. One alternative is to participate in a clinical trial for a new drug candidate; however, these candidates have been exceedingly unsuccessful (more than 99 percent fail), so the probability that a single drug, used alone as a monotherapy, is going to reverse the neurodegenerative process is extremely low, especially since there are typically multiple underlying drivers.

A second alternative is to take a precision medicine approach, determine the root cause and contributors for each person, then address each one. Ultimately, a combination of targeted drugs and personalized programs represents the best hope, but to get there we must "break the envelope," the insistence on single drugs that

ignore the cause of the disease. In order to take this precision medicine approach, we need to understand what factors are driving the
neurodegenerative process in each disease, and beyond that, for
each person. This is where the research informs us.

What our thirty years of research on the neurodegenerative
process taught us led to a new theory: the Mismatch Theory, a
unified theory of neurodegeneration. Here is how this works. For
each functional network of the brain, there are supplies and demands, and these vary from site to site. You've already read about
some of the supplies necessary for the production and maintenance of synapses—the plasticity—that is affected in the disease
of chronic insufficiency we call Alzheimer's disease, such as trophic factors, hormones, nutrients, energy, and insulin sensitivity.
Other functional units of the brain require different supplies, and
of course there is some overlap. On the other side of the equation,
each region has its own demands, based on the requirements for
neuronal activity, structural repair, and maintenance. Thus each
region displays a unique balance of supplies and demands. The
chronic or repeated mismatch between supply and demand—i.e.,
the failure of the supply to keep up with the demand—results in
the neurodegenerative process, a programmatic downsizing that
represents an attempt to realign the demand with the supply
available.

If a theory is accurate, then not only should it be compatible
with published data from different fields such as epidemiology and
biochemistry, but it should also make accurate predictions, such
as how to prevent, halt, or reverse the problem. Let's test out the
Mismatch Theory with an example. There is one neurodegenerative disease that is actually more common than Alzheimer's
disease—about 11 million Americans suffer from it, twice the

number of Alzheimer's patients, and about 170 million globally—and that is age-related macular degeneration (ARMD). ARMD is the leading cause of untreatable visual loss in patients over 50.

The macula is the part of your retina, which sits at the back of your eyes, that is responsible for your accurate central vision, and it is like a Ferrari moving at 200 miles per hour all of the time: it is the most metabolically active part of your body. Any time light is hitting your eyes, your two maculae (one in each eye) are active, and this requires not only a tremendous amount of energy but also active trash removal: the very cells that are responding to the light—photoreceptors—discard their own heads each day (and grow new ones!), filled with trash that is gobbled up by their supporting cells, called retinal pigment epithelial (RPE) cells. This is a bit like the 200-mile-per-hour Ferrari needing frequent oil changes to keep things running cleanly and smoothly. Therefore, anything that increases demand—such as too much high-energy light (blue or purple light) or living near the equator (with more intense sunlight)—increases the risk for macular degeneration. Similarly, anything that reduces the supplies needed for this intense activity—such as poor oxygenation due to sleep apnea or living at high altitude or smoking cigarettes—also increases risk. Furthermore, this mismatch is directly linked to the very inflammatory response that is associated with macular degeneration.

Thus the theme is the same but the specifics are different for Alzheimer's disease and macular degeneration. Alzheimer's is a disease of neuroplasticity resulting from a mismatch in the synaptic support needed for the highly demanding synaptic modifications required for ongoing dynamic, plastic responses; whereas macular degeneration is a disease of energy insufficiency resulting from a mismatch between the uniquely high demand of the macula and the limitations imposed on supply by reduced oxygenation, reduced blood flow, inflammation, toxins (just as dementogens may contribute to cognitive decline, anopsogens may contribute to vision loss), nutrient deficiency, or other factors. Thus macular degeneration is not about plasticity, growth, or constant change; instead it is about a nearly constant, very high demand. In both cases, however, increasing supply and reducing demand represent a rational approach for both prevention and mollification, and in both cases the armamentarium to accomplish this is large and specific to the underlying drivers.

In an analogous fashion, Parkinson's disease has been shown repeatedly to be associated with an energetic failure of one specific part of the mitochondria, a set of proteins directly involved with energy production called complex I. Anything that inhibits this complex—such as the insecticide paraquat or the insecticide/piscicide rotenone or the street drug impurity MPTP—may lead to Parkinson's disease. This indicates that motor modulation—the fine tuning that is lost in Parkinson's—is critically dependent on optimal mitochondrial function, more so than any other system in the body. It is not surprising, therefore, that the response to insufficiency in this system is to slow down, losing the fine tuning and thus developing a slow, unsteady gait, poor balance, and a tremor that reveals a lack of stability at rest.

Parkinson's is typically associated with chemical toxicity, not from dementogens or anopsogens, but from tremorogens. Thus Alzheimer's disease represents a trophic mismatch, macular degeneration a metabolic mismatch, and Parkinson's a mitochondrial energetic mismatch. Optimizing the prevention and treatment of Parkinson's disease therefore involves identifying the mitochondrial toxins present for each person, detoxifying, and providing support for the system involved (the nigrostriatal system of dopaminergic neurons), with targeted trophic factors (GDNF), neurotransmitter support (dopamine precursors such as those found in *Mucuna pruriens*), a plant-rich ketogenic diet (KetoFLEX 12/3), resolving inflammation and removing inflammagens, exercise, treating sleep apnea (and optimizing nocturnal oxygenation), gut healing, probiotics and prebiotics, mitochondrial support, and in appropriate cases, stem cells.

ALS (amyotrophic lateral sclerosis), also called Lou Gehrig's disease, is another motor disease and thus a "cousin" to Parkinson's, but instead of affecting the fine tuning of movement, it affects strength itself, since the motor neurons running directly from brain to spinal cord—the upper motor neurons—and those running from spinal cord to muscles—the lower motor neurons—degenerate in ALS, thus leaving the striated muscles without neural input for voluntary movement. Once again there is a mismatch, and in this case it is something like being on cocaine for years—the neurons essentially dance themselves to death. This phenomenon is called *excitotoxicity*. The neurons are stimulated and excited by the neurotransmitter glutamate, which is wonderful as long as the stimulation is limited by rapid inactivation (which is accomplished by the neurons' supporting cells, the glial cells, which take up the glutamate rapidly and convert it to harmless glutamine). However, if the glutamate is not removed rapidly, the neurons become overstimulated and exhausted, and they die. Talk about too much of a good thing! Thus anything that has the net effect of increasing the glutamate signaling may increase risk for ALS—from being exposed to glutamate-like toxins to compromising the removal system to extending the glutamate release (such as occurs with a seizure) to removing the glutamate-clearing cells to enhancing the glutamate signaling inside the neurons. As an example, research scientist Paul Cox and his team discovered that exposure to a glutamate-mimicking molecule called L-BMAA (L-beta-methylamino alanine) is associated with the development of ALS in people in Guam. It turned out that the source of the L-BMAA was fruit bats, which are a delicacy in Guam, and the fruit bats concentrate the L-BMAA after eating cycad seeds that contain L-BMAA. Beyond Guam, however, many of us globally may also be exposed to L-BMAA, not because we eat fruit bats (most of us don't) but because we are exposed to cyanobacteria, a type of bacterium that produces L-BMAA, which typically lives in lakes.

Fortunately, Dr. Cox and his colleagues have developed a potential treatment for L-BMAA exposure, which is now in clinical trials. This is called L-serine, and, taken at very high doses of up to 30 grams per day, it competes with the L-BMAA, thus reducing the excitotoxicity. Since we don't yet know how many cases of ALS are indeed due to L-BMAA exposure, and since there may be many other contributors, it may take more than L-serine to treat ALS successfully; nonetheless, it is a promising approach, and hopefully the trials will be successful.

As I mentioned, you can arrive at the same place—too much glutamate effect—by several paths, whether it's by adding a mimic like L-BMAA or interfering with the clearance or by another mechanism. There is one toxin to which virtually all of us are exposed, and it increases glutamate by multiple mechanisms: that toxin is glyphosate, and it is on most of our crops and already resides in most of our bodies. Glyphosate increases the amount of glutamate released from our neurons *and* reduces its clearance *and* reduces the detox process itself. Furthermore, glyphosate has an antibacterial effect, altering your gut microbiome and increasing gut leakiness, thus releasing the bacterial component LPS (lipopolysaccharide) into your circulation, which enhances glutamate toxicity, so these multiple effects of glyphosate represent quite a potentially dangerous combination.

There are many other risk factors for ALS, such as lead exposure, statin use, DDT, low testosterone, jobs in power plants or the military, exposure to solvents or radiation, increased zinc levels, copper deficiency, some chronic infections, as well as others. Therefore, an optimal program for ALS might include detoxification (for metals, organics, and biotoxins), increasing glutathione, removal of exposure to identified toxins, gut healing, probiotics and prebiotics, glutamate inhibition, identification and treatment of chronic pathogens, trophic support for motor neurons, liver support (the liver shows damage as a "fatty liver" in over 70 percent of patients with ALS), reduction of homocysteine, discontinuation of statins if possible, hormone optimization, exogenous ketones, reduction in amino acid intake, and antioxidant protection. As for other neurodegenerative diseases, stem cells—for example, adipose-derived stem cells—may also prove valuable.

So how do we go about translating the theory of each neurodegenerative disease and the great amount of information that has been amassed from epidemiological, genetic, pathological, toxicological, microbiological, immunological, and other basic studies into a practical and effective personalized program of treatment? This is where the concept of the PRP—the patient-researcher partnership—comes into play as a highly efficient and effective mechanism. Indeed, the idea of biohacking—changing your own biochemistry with specific supplements, diet, exercise, or other things that "hack the system"—has been around for years, and many nonmedical personnel have undertaken their own treatment for numerous diseases, antiaging effects, cognitive enhancement, and other conditions. In a field in which there is no effective treatment, and in which drug trials have failed repeatedly, such "citizen scientists" and "citizen doctors" may identify novel approaches that complement ongoing research efforts, and indeed there are numerous examples of anecdotal success in cases of neurodegenerative diseases (see, for example, those in healingals.org).

Beyond biohacking, however, partnering researchers with those interested in biohacking and in need of treatment or prevention where none exists in the current standard of care offers more guided biohacking, and has already proven successful in the treatment of cognitive decline, as attested to by some of the survivors' stories in this book. Therefore, those interested in biohacking, in situations in which the standard of care has nothing effective to offer, may consider partnering with insightful researchers—and these may be basic researchers, clinical researchers, or other knowledgeable individuals—to optimize treatment and prevention in a financially efficient manner. This is the goal of the upcoming Ark Project: just as Noah's ark carried individuals two by two by two, the Ark Project seeks to identify a very small number of individuals who are very early in the process of otherwise untreatable neurodegenerative illnesses such as ALS or Lewy body disease or macular degeneration. The plan is then to measure the many potential drivers of the process (the various toxins, metabolic changes, nutrients, pathogens, etc., that are compatible with each pathophysiological process), and address these, iterating to determine whether an initial effective treatment can be devised. Ultimately, this same approach could be applied to many other complex chronic illnesses, such as schizophrenia, autism spectrum disorders, developmental disorders, and lupus, just to name a few.

You can readily see that the landscape for our understanding the neurodegenerative process and fashioning effective treatment and prevention is changing dramatically. What has for over a hundred years been a lack of understanding of the root causes of these "hopeless" illnesses, what has been repeated failure with mono-therapeutic, single-drug approaches, what has been the standard of care, failing to perform the very tests required to determine the mechanisms driving each illness, is finally beginning to give way to a more rational and scientific approach, an evaluation of human patients as highly complex systems with complex network malfunctions often due to several alterations—from toxins and/or pathogens and/or immune activation and/or living outside our evolutionary design, etc.—with more targeted testing, earlier intervention, personalized programs, and iterative optimization. It is a fundamentally different type of medicine—twenty-first-century medicine—one that has moved the entire field of neurodegenerative disease treatment from hopeless to clearly feasible. The results presented by the patients in chapters 1 through 7 prove the success of this new approach.

CHAPTER 12

Gums, Germs, and Steal:
A Pandemic Twofer

Americans will always do the right thing,
after exhausting all the alternatives.
—WINSTON CHURCHILL

opefully, by the time this book is published in the latter
half of 2021, the COVID-19 pandemic will be a thing of
the past. Wishful thinking, I realize. The COVID-19 pandemic is projected to cause the deaths of hundreds of thousands of
Americans, perhaps even a million. For comparison, of the currently living Americans, nearly *fifty times* that many will die of
Alzheimer's disease. So, as widespread as COVID-19 has been, its
numbers are dwarfed by those of the Alzheimer's disease pandemic. To be sure, COVID-19 is a much more acute illness,
whereas Alzheimer's disease is a chronic illness, typically not even
diagnosed until twenty years after the first pathological changes
occur. However, there are remarkable parallels between these two
pandemics, and each has a great deal to teach us about the other.
What's more, the factors predicting poor outcomes in COVID-19

are remarkably similar to those predicting a poor outcome in cognitive decline—truly a pandemic twofer. As Dr. Jeffrey Bland has pointed out, COVID-19 is a pandemic within a pandemic—an infectious pandemic within the pandemic of metabolic disease that has crippled American health for the past several decades. But the origins of these two pandemics have been controversial, as you'll see below.

Fascinating research on the origin of the COVID-19 virus, SARS-CoV-2, by two scientists, Dr. Jonathan Latham and Dr. Allison Wilson, began by asking whether an extraordinary coincidence was truly a coincidence at all. Why did the outbreak of COVID-19 occur within a few hundred yards of the major laboratory that performs extensive research on the very virus that caused the outbreak? This is like investigating an unexplained nuclear explosion that occurred next door to a nuclear test site and concluding that it was a coincidence that had nothing to do with the test site. Sure, it *could* be a coincidence, but it would have been much easier to believe if the COVID-19 outbreak had started in Shanghai or New York or Rome or your brother-in-law's front yard or *anywhere else in the world* other than this specific neighborhood of Wuhan. Occurring as it did in Wuhan, the odds against pure coincidence are astronomical. As Latham and Wilson pointed out, not only is the Wuhan laboratory the major coronavirus research laboratory, and not only have viruses been released in past accidents, but the two viral sequences that resemble SARS-CoV-2 most closely—nearly 99 percent identical—were both being studied in the Wuhan laboratory!

Even more interesting is the source of these nearly identical, closest relatives of SARS-CoV-2. These were sent to the Wuhan laboratory from a mine in Mojiang, China, a mine filled with, you guessed it, bats and bat guano. While removing the bat excrement in 2012, six miners fell ill with a disease that is a dead ringer— literally, unfortunately—for COVID-19. Multiple samples were taken from these miners, three of whom died, and delivered to the Wuhan lab, but could not be studied in the lab (and thus were safely frozen away) until a "secure" BSL-4 (biosafety level 4, the highest biosafety level) facility was built for such virus studies, delaying the research until 2018. Then in 2019, bingo, a "mysterious" new illness, COVID-19, appeared just outside the lab, and spread to every corner of the world, killing millions in the process. Coincidence? Maybe.

The origins of dementia go much further back, of course, and although Dr. Alois Alzheimer did not provide his classic description of the pathology of what came to be called Alzheimer's disease until 1906, dementia was described in antiquity by Ayurvedic physicians, as well as by the Greeks and Romans. However, with increases in type 2 diabetes, prediabetes, obesity, and systemic inflammation over the past several decades, Alzheimer's has risen to become the third leading cause of death in the United States.

The interrelationship of these two superficially dissimilar diseases is remarkable. COVID-19 has compressed the risk factors that operate over decades in Alzheimer's disease into just a few weeks, but they are strikingly similar: those with type 2 diabetes, those with prediabetes, those with obesity, those with hypertension and vascular disease, those with an increased tendency to blood clotting, those with advanced age, those with deficiency of vitamin D, those with deficiency of zinc, those with the genetic risk factor ApoE4, those with weakened adaptive immune systems, can all expect a poorer outcome from COVID-19 and are all at greater risk for Alzheimer's disease. In a corollary fashion, correcting these same metabolic and physiological parameters reduces risk for poor outcomes in COVID-19 and reduces risk for the development of Alzheimer's disease.

Arguably the most important cause of mortality in COVID-19 is a cytokine storm, the runaway inflammation often treated with the anti-inflammatory steroid dexamethasone. Part of this same response—the inflammation associated with the innate immune system, the evolutionarily older part of our immune systems—is the amyloid we associate with Alzheimer's disease! The very stuff that collects in our brains when we develop Alzheimer's, the stuff we have vilified as the cause of Alzheimer's, the stuff that the drugs like aducanumab get rid of, is part of our immune system's attempt to deal with insults such as viral or bacterial infections! So in some ways, Alzheimer's is like a decades-long, very mild cytokine storm—more like a cytokine drizzle, actually—and thus the key is to identify and treat the chronic infections (or other insults) that are driving the process—such as leaky gut, gingivitis ("leaky gums"), periodontitis (inflammation around the teeth), or sinusitis—*then* remove the amyloid. Just removing the amyloid without removing the insults would be like giving a COVID-19 patient dexamethasone while continuing to expose him/her to more virus day after day! Not a very rational strategy.

You may have seen an interesting documentary series entitled *The Food That Built America*, which describes the origins of iconic foods such as Heinz Ketchup, Kellogg's Corn Flakes, Coca-Cola, Hershey's Milk Chocolate, and McDonald's burgers. It is fascinating to hear how these various foods were developed and popularized. But at the heart of nearly all of the foods that built America—the delicious factor that made them billion-sellers—is sugar. Sugar in fast food, sugar in processed food, sugar in fun food, sugar in canned food, sugar in condiments for food. As the old song goes, "sugar in the mornin', sugar in the evenin', sugar at suppertime"—and every other mealtime. Sugar—The Food That Built America is also The Food That Devastated America. The insulin resistance that drives Alzheimer's risk and COVID-19 mortality risk, the metabolic syndrome, the hypertension, the obesity, the early aging, the vascular disease, the leptin resistance, the chronic illnesses and early mortality, the ubiquitous cognitive decline, and the overwhelming death toll from COVID-19. We humans were simply not designed evolutionarily to consume the amounts of sugar that we are exposed to, and we are paying for it with our health. Sugar has become our number one dementogen, the most common brain stealer, and a critical risk factor in COVID-19 mortality risk.

But hey, for those who have already recovered from COVID-19, you are out of the woods, right? Would that it were so. Many are left with brain fog, trouble concentrating, chronic fatigue, shortness of breath, headache, muscle pain, palpitations, anosmia (loss of the sense of smell), ageusia (loss of the sense of taste), insomnia, rashes, or hair loss—all parts of what has been referred to as "long haulers syndrome." How long these symptoms may last is as yet unknown. But a much larger issue looms on the horizon: a few case reports of relatively young patients developing Parkinson's disease immediately after COVID-19 have now appeared, reminding us all of the nearly 1 million cases of Parkinson's that occurred after epidemic viral illness a century ago. Are Alzheimer's and Parkinson's the future of COVID-19? For the over 100 million people who have developed COVID-19 globally, this is a long-term concern, and a reason to be on a prevention protocol.

Meanwhile, hopefully the vaccines will protect the billions at risk, and hopefully improved anti-coronavirals will become available, since remdesivir has shown little efficacy. However, it is clear that resilience, optimal immune function, and optimal metabolic function are highly effective strategies both for prevention of COVID-19 and for cognitive decline.

The United States has suffered far more deaths due to COVID-19 than any other country, and while some of this is likely to be related to high-risk behavior, it is also likely to reflect our metabolic health as a country—yet another factor in common with Alzheimer's disease risk. COVID-19 has brought home the seriousness of our chronic ill health, as well as increasing anxiety, isolation, depression, and insomnia. However, in so doing, it is spurring all of us on to focus on improving our metabolic health, immune health, and overall resilience.

CHAPTER 13

Enhancing "Normal" Cognition: Be All You Can Be

What the world needs is more geniuses with humility.
There are so few of us left.

—OSCAR LEVANT

I'm good enough, I'm smart enough,
and doggone it, people like me.

—STUART SMALLEY (FORMER SENATOR AL FRANKEN),
SATURDAY NIGHT LIVE

Doctors used to believe that a person was either diabetic or not diabetic. Even the diabetes experts subscribed to this notion. Just like pregnancy, either you were or you weren't. Now, of course, we know that long before diabetes is diagnosed, prediabetes occurs, along with the associated insulin resistance, so there is a spectrum of high blood sugar and its related metabolic damage, leading ultimately to diabetes.

The same misunderstanding happened with Alzheimer's: it used to be believed that "normal" cognition preceded Alzheimer's disease, and there was no designation for what lay in between. Thankfully, our view is now much more nuanced than that. I say *thankfully* because it is the long stage of pre-Alzheimer's that offers us the most immediate opportunity for complete reversals of cognitive decline, as we have seen and documented repeatedly. The journey from normal cognition to Alzheimer's disease may take twenty years or so, and that means there is a huge window of opportunity to intervene.

But what about "normalcy"? Just as there is a long period of milder impairment that precedes obvious, diagnosed Alzheimer's, for many of us our ostensibly "normal" cognition is actually operating well below its full potential. This is true not just for people who are on the path to Alzheimer's; nearly every one of us could enhance our cognitive abilities. In fact, the whole concept of "normal" is a bit scary these days: the "normal" American has hypertension, hypercholesterolemia, insulin resistance; is overweight; has a leaky gut; is on at least one prescription medication (and 20 percent of us are on five or more); is likely taking a statin and/or an antihypertensive and/or a proton pump inhibitor; is deficient in zinc, magnesium, selenium, and iodine; and is highly unlikely to manifest optimal cognition!

We all are compromised (some more than others, but all of us to some extent) by factors such as flawed dietary and lifestyle choices, suboptimal sleep, unrecognized exposure to chemotoxins (including air pollution) and biotoxins, microbiomes that aren't what they could be, suboptimal brain stimulation, hidden pathogens, some degree of ongoing inflammation, suboptimal cerebral blood flow, suboptimal oxygenation, and numerous other suboptimal factors, each playing on the background of our personal genome and epigenome. Just as we are coming to realize that most of us are suboptimal in our metabolism—burdened with insulin resistance, a less-than-ideal lipid profile, clogged detoxification pathways, unbalanced gut microbiome, and so forth—we are increasingly coming to realize that the vast majority of us are also walking around with a "normal" cognition that is far from our best.

It may not sound like it, but this is good news, too. If your current cognition is less than optimal—which is the case for virtually every one of us—then there is room to improve it. And since we are nearly all working with suboptimal brains, we all have an opportunity to become sharper.

After all, cognition is arguably the most important and essential human quality. The difference between "normal" cognition and superior cognition is the difference between the status quo and innovation, between increasing problems and finding solutions, between failure and success. Therefore, enhancing "normal" cognition has far-reaching implications—for improved work, better mood, fewer accidents, fewer mistakes, better ideas, and an overall richer and more successful life. This applies to everyone, from 20-somethings to 90-somethings (and beyond!). Essentially we are coming to a new realization of what "to be healthy" actually means, as our tests are more extensive and mechanistically based. We can now determine our levels of health, risk, and function like never before, and improve them, with remarkable impact on everything from cognition to the immune system to many age-associated diseases.

Cam is a 49-year-old man whose wife suffered cognitive decline and began the protocol, which he adopted in support right along with her. Although he had no cognitive complaints, over the next several months he lost twenty pounds and noticed a clear improvement in energy, an enhanced mood, better focus, and an improved memory. His performance at work improved so markedly that his younger coworkers began to ask him what he had been doing.

All of the tools you have read about up to this point—the KetoFLEX 12/3 diet, the techniques for managing stress, exercise, and improving sleep, all of it—applies to you. It will all help you live a better life, and it will fine-tune your cognition no matter what your current state is. In that sense, this entire book is about enhancing cognition. In this chapter, though, we will go further. Here we explore the vast armamentarium that is available to all of us—from effects on neurotransmitters to second messengers to synaptic structure to trophic factors to mitochondrial energy, and dozens of other targets—that can elevate your brain to a new, higher "normal."

What we are talking about here is very different from the short-term boosts (you can think of them as improvised brain hacks) that many people turn to when they need a mental lift. Drugs like Adderall or cocaine or amphetamines do their work and then they are gone—or worse. They can lead to addiction and negative, even devastating side effects. We are seeking out a healthier and more sustainable type of enhancement: the kind of long-term improvement that can be realized with increased cholinergic support, increased BDNF, optimized hormones, and optimized gut microbiome, among many other parameters. A properly enhanced brain is one that should *stay* enhanced as part of a sustainable, balanced lifestyle. This approach requires more effort than popping a pill, but it will produce the kind of change you really want.

What does it take to support memory and overall cognition?

There is an old neuroscience principle: "neurons that fire together, wire together," meaning that repeated association of input with output strengthens the circuit. In practical terms, this means that repetition will aid in the creation and maintenance of memories, whether these memories are for learning a new language or the use of a new smartphone or a new musical instrument or any of many other learned tasks or information. When we do this learning, we want to optimize all of the contributors, just as when you are building a house you want to have the right blueprints, the best workers, the highest-quality building materials, the proper permits, and so on. So let's have a look at how we can best build our "house of memories."

In order to create and maintain the synaptic connections that we need to form and retain memories, we'll want to establish the proper brain chemistry to support both the wiring and the firing. That may sound simple, but your brain depends on a highly complex system of supplies. There are neurotransmitters, chemicals that mediate the signals between neurons. There are neurotrophins, which nourish your neurons and support the formation of new synapses, semipermanent linkages from neuron to neuron. There is axoplasmic transport, a multistage process that shuttles cell parts and molecular resources along the axon, the long "tail" of a neuron that carries electrical signals through the brain. And that's just the beginning. Other systems minimize inflammatory signaling and regulate mitochondrial membrane potential and function, metal homeostasis, protein folding, the function of supporting cells such as astrocytes and microglia, myelination (the fatty insulation wrapped around neurons), and numerous other parameters critical for optimized brain function.

All of this activity supports 100 billion brain cells that make about 500 trillion connections. And yet compared to a modern digital computer, the brain's processing speed is quite modest, just 60 bits per second by one measure. The human brain utilizes its resources very differently than a computer does, but they have one fundamental similarity: faster processing means more power. Brain training is helpful to make the most of those 60 bits per second. Antiaging techniques are also important, since the brain's processing speed and its number of active connections are closely linked to biological age.

HOW TO BUILD AND SUSTAIN A BETTER BRAIN

Step one of enhancing your brain is enacting the fundamental protocols we have outlined for preventing cognitive decline: a clean diet, abundant exercise, high-quality sleep, and avoidance of chronic stress (in contrast, acute stress with resolution is not nearly as damaging, and may actually be supportive, a process called hormesis). In addition, brain-training programs are both fun and useful for honing your thought process. BrainHQ is the program with the most scientific support, and this includes many programs for memory, processing speed, executive function, and other cognitive skills. Other options include Elevate, Dakim BrainFitness, and Lumosity, among others. For many people, especially the teenagers, 20-somethings, and 30-somethings, these actions may be enough. You can tell based on a cognoscopy—blood tests that evaluate the critical parameters for cognition and cognitive risk, coupled with an easy online cognitive screen such as CNS Vital Signs or

Cogstate. There is increased risk after age 40 for the very factors that impede optimal cognition, so more aggressive interventions may be called for.

Such interventions are now possible because we can study and monitor ourselves as never before. As our tests become more extensive and mechanistically based, we are coming to a new realization of what it actually means "to be healthy." No longer do we need to be satisfied with the negative definition of health as "not ill" or "not impaired." We can now determine our level of health like never before, compare it to what it could be, and improve it. This targeted, data-driven approach is having a remarkable impact on everything from the immune system to many age-associated diseases—and of course it is having an impact on cognition as well.

Step two of enhancing your brain involves enlisting a personalized array of nootropic (cognitive-enhancing) agents, many of which have multiple mechanisms of action. We have outlined some of the major ones here. As with ReCODE, you will want to test, tweak, and adjust your personal protocol as you discover how your own brain responds.

A Brain-Enhancing Pharmacopoeia

- **Enhancing neurotransmission by acetylcholine:** This neurotransmitter is critical for conveying messages between and from neurons. Supplements that may assist its work include huperzine A (derived from Chinese club moss, *Huperzia serrata*), *Bacopa monnieri* (also known as brahmi, a traditional Indian medicinal plant), citicoline, alpha-GPC, and lecithin, an essential fat found in many foods, including eggs.

• **Enhancing cyclic AMP:** Adenosine monophosphate (AMP) is an important messenger for brain plasticity. Caffeine, an adenosine inhibitor, boosts cyclic AMP, as does L-theanine, an amino acid found in tea and certain mushrooms.

• **Optimizing glutamatergic vs. GABAergic transmission:** Glutamate is the most common neurotransmitter in the body. Gamma-aminobutyric acid (GABA) suppresses excess signaling by neurons. An overabundance of glutamate over GABA is associated with anxiety, depression, restlessness, inability to concentrate, headaches, insomnia, fatigue, and increased sensitivity to pain. You can restore balance with valerian (a medicinal root extract), vitamin B_6, and lemon balm, and by taking GABA directly.

• **Supporting mitochondrial function:** Mitochondria are the energy production units (organelles) inside the cells of your body. They are critical to cognition and indeed to all metabolism. Endogenous ketones, derived from breaking down your adipose tissue, are converted to acetyl-CoA and metabolized by mitochondria. Exogenous ketones (such as ketone salts or esters) also provide energy, but lack some of the advantages of endogenous ketones, such as the associated anti-inflammatory effect.

The goal is to create metabolic flexibility, so that your mitochondria can metabolize either carbohydrates or fats/ketones.

Useful supplements include ubiquinol (also sold as Coenzyme Q10, or CoQ10), PQQ (pyrroloquinoline quinone, which increases mitochondrial number), R-lipoic acid (an antioxidant and enabling molecule also found in spinach and broccoli), ALCAR (acetyl-L-carnitine, a metabolism-supporting amino acid), creatine (which provides energy), and nicotinamide riboside—a form of vitamin B3 that increases NAD+ (nicotinamide adenine dinucleotide). As noted in chapter 10, methylene blue holds promise as another method to enhance mitochondrial function.

- **Supporting neurotransmission by dopamine:** In the brain, dopamine is a primary signaling molecule that is especially associated with the "reward" pathway that reinforces certain behaviors; loss of dopamine-producing cells contributes to Parkinson's disease. Supplements that may aid dopamine production include tyrosine and phenylalanine (two essential amino acids), and vitamin B6.

- **Supporting synaptic structure:** A healthy brain depends on a robust cellular infrastructure. To help maintain the physical condition of your neurons, try citicoline and its chemical relative, alpha-GPC (glycerylphosphorylcholine), as well as DHA (docosahexaenoic acid), an omega-3 fatty acid also found in fish, especially cold-water fish.

• **Improving mental focus:** Supplements that may help sharpen your thinking include gotu kola (a traditional Chinese and Ayurvedic herb), shankhpushpi (an Ayurvedic medicine), and pantothenic acid (vitamin B5). Many people report success from therapeutic hot/cold treatment, alternating between a hot sauna and cold water to stimulate the sensory response and also enhance mitochondrial function.

• **Enhancing brain-derived neurotrophic factor (BDNF):** This essential protein promotes the formation and maintenance of neurons in the body. You can boost your BDNF with whole coffee fruit extract (WCFE) and dihydroxyflavones (7,8-DHF). There is also a simple and pleasurable technique that boosts BDNF while providing many other physical and psychological benefits—exercise—and there are some enhancements of exercise, such as EWOT (exercise with oxygen therapy) and KAATSU (which uses bands to increase the physiological response to exercise), which may boost exercise advantages.

• **Enhancing nerve-growth factor (NGF):** Along with BNDF, NGF is critical to the growth, maintenance, and survival of nerve cells. NGF-promoting supplements include *Hericium erinaceus* (lion's mane mushroom), ALCAR, and specific strains of bacteria in the gut microbiome (e.g., some bifidobacteria), which can be boosted by taking probiotics.

• **Enhancing sirtuin 1 (SIRT1):** Recent research indicates that this protein stimulates autophagy and provokes an antiaging response in laboratory animals. It is being explored more broadly as an antiaging mediator, and it also enhances the synaptoblastic (anti-Alzheimer's) signaling of the amyloid precursor protein, APP. You can increase SIRT1 function by taking resveratrol (found in grapes and red wine, but also in many berries), nicotinamide riboside, NMN (nicotinamide mononucleotide, a derivative of niacin), and NAD+. You can also stimulate your body's production of NAD+ with exercise and fasting.

• **Promoting blood flow:** Ginkgo has been shown to increase blood flow by stimulating production of nitric oxide, which dilates the blood vessels. Nitric oxide can also be increased by L-arginine, Neo40, beetroot extract, and arugula.

• **Improving mood:** In some cases, you can go straight to the desired effect—and do it without the common drugs that have significant side effects. Saffron is a natural antidepressant; it appears to work by increasing serotonin levels. Lemon balm has also been shown to be effective.

• **Reducing chronic stress:** Acute stress, with resolution, is something we all deal with, and it does not impede cognition. However, the unrelenting chronic stress that so many of us experience is associated with brain atrophy. There are many methods to address this, from meditation to yoga to social interactions (admittedly more difficult during the pandemic) to music to shinrin-yoku (the Japanese technique of "forest bathing"), and others—whatever brings you joy, relaxation, and fulfillment.

- **Optimizing methylation:** Methylcobalamin (Me-B12, a form of vitamin B12), pyridoxal-5'-phosphate (P5P, an active form of vitamin B6), and methylfolate (another B-complex vitamin) all regulate methylation, which is critical for the epigenome and its readout of specific genes, as well as for detoxification, among other processes.

- **Minimizing inflammation and supporting adaptive immunity:** As we've noted previously, inflammation is strongly linked with cognitive decline. Many supplements can help you control inflammation and the effects that come with it. Curcumin (derived from turmeric), ginger, and *Withania somnifera* (ashwagandha from Ayurvedic medicine) all have been shown to be effective. As noted in chapter 10, it is also important to resolve any ongoing inflammation, which can be accomplished with specialized pro-resolving mediators (SPMs) or high-dose omega-3 fats (2 to 4 grams), and to remove the source of inflammation, whether it be from a leaky gut, metabolic syndrome, chronic infections, or another source. LDN (low-dose naltrexone) is also helpful for optimizing immune function and reducing inflammation.

  Supporting adaptive immunity includes optimizing zinc (and this is a very common deficiency), vitamin D, and considering quercetin, R-lipoic acid, and AHCC (active hexose correlated compound).

- **Enhancing detox, minimizing toxin levels:** There are many paths to reducing the toxin load in your body, as noted in chapter 10, and we developed PreCODE for optimizing prevention of cognitive decline. Finding and eliminating sources of toxin exposure is essential, of course. Sulforaphane (found in cabbage and broccoli), glutathione (a common antioxidant), and N-acetyl cysteine (NAC) help cleanse the body. Eating a high-fiber diet and drinking filtered water will aid you in eliminating toxins. An infrared sauna followed by cleansing with castile soap can also be effective.

- **Healing your gut:** An increasing wealth of research has shown unequivocally that your body's microbial ecosystem is essential to your physical and mental health. The KetoFLEX 12/3 lifestyle incorporates multiple techniques for optimizing your microbiome, including eating a diet rich in fermented foods, plant proteins, and fiber. Reducing your toxin load and minimizing antibiotics and microbiome-suppressing drugs like proton pump inhibitors (PPIs) are also important.

- **Optimizing nutrient status:** Beyond the individual supplements, you should strive for overall nutritional balance in your diet. Note, for example, that cognition is better with high-normal levels of vitamin B_{12} than with mid-normal or low-normal levels. There is an extensive discussion on optimal brain nutrition in *The End of Alzheimer's Program*.

• **Optimizing antioxidant status:** The widespread idea that more antioxidants are preferable is overly simplistic. In reality, you need *both* oxidant and antioxidant effects, in optimal balance. Depending on your personal biochemistry, you may need to boost your levels of vitamin E, glutathione, vitamin C, sulforaphane, ubiquinol, vinpocetine (a synthetic version of a drug found in periwinkle), and SkQ and mitoquinol (which target the mitochondria).

• **Fasting:** Fasting has numerous salutary effects, from enhancing ketosis to improving glycemic control and supporting insulin sensitivity to improving lipid status to improving blood pressure to enhancing autophagy and mitophagy, among others. Thus fasting is the base of the brain food pyramid (at least twelve hours between the end of supper and the start of breakfast or lunch, and at least three hours between supper and bedtime). The earlier in life you begin fasting, the longer and more thoroughly you will reap the benefits.

• **Monitoring:** As noted in chapter 10, we all now have access to numerous tracking tools, for everything from blood oxygen to ketone level to sleep quality and quantity to heart rate variation, and many others. To tweak your enhancement protocol, you will want to pay special attention to your blood oxygen levels (using the Apple

Watch or the iPhone or Beddr or another oximeter), heart rate variability (using the Apple Watch or the Oura ring), ketone levels (using the Biosense breathalyzer or the Precision Xtra or the Keto-Mojo ketone meter), glucose levels (using continuous glucose monitoring or the Precision Xtra glucose meter), sleep quality and quantity (using the Oura ring or the Apple Watch), nutrients (using the Cronometer website), exercise timing (using any of the many wearables such as a Fitbit or the Apple Watch), and vascular elasticity (using iHeart).

• **Optimizing hormonal status:** For most of us, optimizing our diet, exercise, sleep, stress level, and microbiome will allow us to produce highly functional levels of hormones such as estradiol, testosterone, progesterone, pregnenolone, and DHEA. However, for others, whether due to autoimmunity (for example, Hashimoto's thyroiditis, which results in reduced thyroid levels) or toxicity or simple carbohydrates or other causes, one or more hormones will be reduced, which can affect cognition. Returning these to optimal with the help of a functional endocrinologist or internist can often help to enhance cognition.

• **Oral health and microbiome:** Organisms from the oral microbiome are showing up, quite remarkably, in the brain, in atherosclerotic lesions, and even in cancers, suggesting that there is widespread communication of these organisms throughout the body, including effects on the brain and thus cognition. Optimizing your oral microbiome starts with checking OralDNA testing for pathogens such as *P. gingivalis, T. denticola, F. nucleatum,* and *P. intermedia.* If you find that you have significant levels of these pathogens, you can improve your oral microbiome with Dentalcidin toothpaste and mouthwash, followed by a probiotic toothpaste such as Revitin. If you have gingivitis or periodontitis, consultation with an oral-systemic specialist is recommended.

• **Functional genomics:** Whole genome sequencing has become very affordable, and this should become standard for any health evaluation in the near future. However, even small fractional genomes, such as the one offered by 23andMe, can be extremely helpful, offering data (with the appropriate evaluation) on ApoE status, Alzheimer's risk, detoxification (and thus risk for toxin-associated illnesses such as dementia), vascular risk, thrombotic tendency, and many other health parameters. Evaluation programs such as Genetic Genie and IntellxxDNA are very helpful for strategizing optimal brain function and overall health.

• **Youth factors:** The interest in "young plasma" (heterochronic parabiosis) for aging individuals is still undergoing substantiation, but one of the interesting follow-up studies showed that the majority of the salutary effects may simply be due to the removal of "aging factors" by plasmapheresis, which would be a much simpler and less expensive alternative. As noted above, renewal and regeneration using stem cells has remarkable potential, and ongoing clinical trials (even though carried out as a mono-therapy, and thus suboptimally) should help to determine the magnitude of effect these may have on cognition.

- **Short-term interventions:** As noted above, short-term hy-peractivation with agents such as amphetamines, co-caine, or Adderall can certainly enhance cognition, but this comes at a price, since long-term effects such as ad-diction, fatigue, and vasculitis may ensue. However, there are safer short-term alternatives such as Nuvigil (which inhibits drowsiness and supports alertness) and the racetams piracetam, aniracetam, and phenylpirace-tam. The racetams have a nootropic effect, improving memory and cognition, and have few short-term side ef-fects, although some people develop insomnia or anxiety. However, these bind to glutamate receptors, and there-fore you may not want to continue them indefinitely; that said, the long-term use has not to date suggested in-creased risk of glutamate-receptor-related conditions such as seizures or ALS, so these nootropics may be very helpful for enhancing memory and overall cognition even on a long-term basis.

- **Coming possibilities:** There are exciting possibilities up-coming, which should continue to advance our ability to enhance cognition: targeted probiotics offer strains that increase specific trophic factors and neurotransmit-ters; evaluation of the microbiomes of organs thought classically to be sterile—such as blood and brain—should

offer new insights into unrecognized organisms impact-
ing cognition (both positively and negatively); CRISPR
will allow gene manipulation, with its clear clinical and
ethical implications; and retinal amyloid imaging should
allow early recognition of amyloid accumulation, which
as noted above begins to occur about twenty years prior
to the diagnosis of Alzheimer's, thus offering an excellent
early warning system.

For most of us, there will be specific reasons that our "normal"
cognition can be enhanced. For some of us, it will be because we
have some degree of insulin resistance, as 80 million Americans
have, and reversing this will improve cognition. For others of us,
it will be suboptimal sleep quantity and/or quality, and optimizing
that will improve cognition. For still others, it will turn out to be
chronic stress, which can be managed effectively. And for others,
it may be mild chronic inflammation from a leaky gut, or too little
exercise, or mild vascular disease, or suboptimal hormone levels,
or dietary choline deficiency or a vitamin D deficiency. Optimizing these critical brain parameters will allow all of us to be sharper
and stay sharper for decades to come.

CHAPTER 14

The Revolution Will Not Be Televised (or Reimbursed)

*Every revolution seems impossible at the beginning,
and after it happens, it was inevitable.*

—BILL AYERS

evolutions are in some ways the human equivalent of earthquakes—massive, deadly tectonic shifts. Of course, in the case of revolutions, the shifts are in ideology and governance, but the death tolls often exceed those from even the largest earthquakes. The American Revolutionary War resulted in the deaths of 37,000 people. The French Revolution, about 40,000. The Mexican Revolution, over 500,000. And the Russian Revolution, somewhere between 5 and 9 million. But these sobering numbers are dwarfed by the number of deaths in the ongoing medical revolution—which is surprising, since most people are unaware that such a revolution is happening at all. Furthermore, whereas in most revolutions, the revolutionaries and the members of the regime in power are the main ones dying in the struggle ("collateral damage" notwithstanding), in the current medical revolution, the casualties are you and me and the many patients—not the revolutionaries or the target regime itself—which, disappointingly, offers much less incentive for the current regime to consider change, no matter how ineffective it is shown to be.

Over a hundred years ago—in 1910—Abraham Flexner presented a landmark report now called the Flexner Report. It is regarded as the bible that shaped the religion of American medical teaching. Its repercussions continue to this day, and its impact is unequaled in American medical education history.

In order to investigate American medical schools, Flexner visited all 155 of those then training students in the United States and was appalled at some of the teaching practices he discovered. Curricula and quality of education varied wildly from school to school, as did entrance requirements. At many schools, the profit motive seemed to outweigh the scholastic one.

Flexner recommended that American medical schools be brought more in line with their European counterparts, with increased focus on the scientific underpinnings of medicine, more rigorous entrance requirements, more hands-on experience, more faculty engaged in research, and increased state regulation of physician licensure. He also recommended that 80 percent of the medical schools be closed (and over 50 percent did end up closing).

There is no question that the Flexner Report improved American medical education dramatically. However, in some ways, it is very much a dated document. For example, it recommended that African American doctors not be allowed to treat Caucasian patients, and that all medical schools historically training African American physicians be closed, save for two. While well intentioned in its recommendations such as more rigorous admissions standards and more patient-oriented training, the Flexner Report was a product of its time, and it imposed constraints in practice that did not anticipate the societal, scientific, and medical advances that have occurred since 1910.

Imagine that Flexner had instead evaluated the airline industry in 1910 (okay, the first commercial flight wasn't until 1914, but you see my point), and recommended that all future airlines fly the most advanced biplanes with the best kick-starting propellers. He would have had no way of anticipating jet travel in 1910, and indeed, in his medical school evaluations, he had no way of anticipating systems biology, big data, the human genome, the internet, telemedicine, or precision medicine.

A CONFEDERACY OF DOCTORS

One need only compare the mercurial progress in software and technology to the unenterprising, century-out-of-date medical training we are now faced with in order to see why we are in the midst of the bloodiest revolution in history. While we still train the physicians who hold our lives in their hands based on a single, unupdated 1910 document, the Apple Watch is now in its sixth iteration. Medical schools are the covered wagons of today—atavistic but so ingrained in our society that they operate unquestioned.

Flexner focused on the methodology—how to train new physicians—instead of on patient outcomes, with the idea that rigorous and uniform training would lead to the best outcomes. However, the methodology that led to best patient outcomes in 1910 is a far cry from what is required today. When would it be appropriate for an update to the 1910 recommendations? Perhaps

1920 would make sense? If so, the updated report is 100 years late. At some point, the lack of an update becomes absurd, and counterproductive to medical training.

One of the common concerns in 1910 was quackery, and with schools admitting unqualified candidates, failing to provide rigorous training, using alternative and unproven therapeutic approaches, and pushing students through simply for profit, it is no wonder that medical quacks abounded. These quacks used ineffective therapeutic approaches and failed to effect patient improvement. The Flexner Report cut back on the medical quackery of 1910, but what should we call it when modern physicians use outdated, ineffective approaches and fail to effect patient improvement, when there are effective therapeutic options available? Shall they, too, be called quacks?

As I mentioned above, when our daughter developed lupus and was evaluated by two international experts, neither of whom had any insight into why she had developed it or what therapy to offer (other than "steroids when it gets worse"), and we then took her to a "functional medicine" physician who determined why she had lupus and was able to treat her successfully (she has been asymptomatic for over ten years now), we wondered: Were these "experts" actually quacks? Was the "alternative medicine" physician actually the expert? Certainly if labels were based solely on patient outcome, those would be fair descriptions.

Beyond lupus, so many of the diseases we studied in medical school are without known cause and/or effective treatment: Alzheimer's disease, Parkinson's disease (for which there is symptomatic treatment only), frontotemporal dementia, Lewy body disease, vascular dementia, ALS (amyotrophic lateral sclerosis), chronic traumatic encephalopathy, progressive supranuclear palsy,

corticobasal degeneration, macular degeneration, autism, schizophrenia, ADD (attention deficit disorder), and many autoimmune and inflammatory disorders such as inflammatory bowel
disease, Sjögren's syndrome, and scleroderma (progressive systemic sclerosis).

Standard-of-care medicine does not identify the underlying
cause(s) of these illnesses, nor does it offer effective treatment. In
contrast, "alternative medicine" physicians such as functional
medicine and integrative medicine physicians focus on root cause
analysis, and targeting root causes often leads to success. Indeed, our research on the molecular mechanisms of Alzheimer's
disease—in which we were agnostic, focusing only on the underlying mechanistic biochemistry—led directly to a therapeutic
approach—ReCODE—that is much more reminiscent of "alternative medicine" than it is of standard allopathic medicine.
This was something not anticipated by the Flexner Report, and
something that was a surprise to me as a classically trained
neurologist.

As Hegel pointed out, thesis and antithesis lead to synthesis,
so these two disparate approaches to medicine should foment
progress, right? Unfortunately, when standard-of-care medicine
has nothing effective to offer for a disease, the response to learning
of an alternative approach that is more effective has not been to
upgrade the standard-of-care approach, but rather to do just the
opposite—use all methods and connections to shut it down. The
healthcare payers will not reimburse (because of course there is no
incentive for them to do so—if you can avoid adding to your coverage list, there will be more profit) despite reimbursing far more
expensive, less effective pharmaceutical approaches; the practicing
physicians are too busy to learn the new approaches; the drug

companies focus on profitable monotherapeutics; and we all suffer from the gargantuan inertia in the system.

If you wanted to set up a system that would *prevent* innovation and novel therapeutics, what would you do? You might focus on philanthropy to drain the finances of those interested in seeing novel approaches, hire consultants who are competing with the potential innovators (and thus anything but impartial), accept support from nonobjective for-profit entities, criticize novel approaches, and support the outdated treatments that have failed repeatedly. In other words, if you wanted to set up a system that would prevent innovation and novel, effective therapeutics, you would be hard pressed to do better than some of our current established foundations.

The excuse for all of this is that the new approach is "unproven," but this is like saying, "I prefer something that I know does not work over hope and at least some success." This is not the response of caring humans. It is the response of misguided egotism and a profit-driven motive, and it is leading to countless unnecessary cases of morbidity and mortality, from dozens of complex chronic diseases.

Years ago, just after finishing my training in neurology, one of my jobs was to evaluate people who were seeking insurance for various neurological conditions. One patient was sent for evaluation because he complained of an inability to walk. Examining him, it was clear to me that there was no neurological reason he could not walk, and I recorded that in my notes. A few weeks later, I received a call from a man identifying himself as a social worker who had been helping the man I had examined. He was calling to warn me that the patient had received a note from the insurance company that denied his claim, quoting my examination and name. The denial made him very angry, and he decided that he was going to kill me, which is why the social worker had called—to let me know that the patient was on his way. Of course, this scared the hell out of me. I asked the social worker, "How is he getting here?" To which he replied, "He's walking."

I was fairly certain that the irony of this was lost on the perambulatory would-be murderer, but I did not want to dwell on that; I wanted to get away from where I thought that he thought I would be. I called the police, who informed me that "There is nothing we can do simply because someone claims he is on his way to kill you. But don't worry, if he succeeds, we'll get him." Great, that was helpful.

Fortunately, the patient ultimately thought better of his plan, and after blowing off some steam, decided not to murder me. Then a few weeks later, I received another call from the social worker—the patient had decided that I had done a good job with my evaluation, I was a good doctor, and would I be his doctor? (No, I'm not making this stuff up.)

As this patient demonstrated, truth can be one of the most dangerous commodities, one that sometimes must be released cautiously. Truth frequently runs counter to consensus, and when it does, woe to him that puts truth ahead of group politics! Maimonides said, "Truth does not become more true by virtue of the fact that the entire world agrees with it, nor less so even if the whole world disagrees with it." However, clearly he was not talking to the medical establishment, or to big pharma, or to healthcare conglomerates.

Last week I received a call from a journalist who told me she had been commissioned to write an article for a medical journal, an article about the "complaints" about the ReCODE Protocol that my colleagues and I had developed. She was calling because as an experienced journalist, she wanted to get both sides of the story, so she was calling to get my version. While I appreciated that—another far less competent journalist had written an article with only one side of the story, a piece that would have earned a failing grade in high school journalism—I thought it strange that the journal had asked for an article focused on complaints in a discussion of the first hope for an otherwise untreatable illness. So let me get this straight: The journal is implying that if someone with cognitive decline goes to a standard clinic and is told there is no hope, he or she should just go home and die—there is no complaint about that? On the other hand, if years of research suggest that there is indeed hope for the first time, and this is documented in multiple publications, with hundreds of people improving—that is something to complain about? Maybe a better way to proceed would be to start by talking with some of the first survivors and ask them about complaints?

What is happening in the field of Alzheimer's therapeutics is a microcosm of what is happening in the field of medicine. There are two competing, fundamentally different approaches, and the lack of synthesis of these approaches is repeatedly harming patients. The revolution, unheralded though it may be, is truly a bloody one.

In medicine, the gap between truth and acceptance is widening, to the detriment of our health. This gap is driven by finances, politics, and influence, and such a widening gap is exactly what drives revolutions. Success will require putting in place policies to minimize this gap on an ongoing basis, focusing on patient outcomes rather than outdated reports or drug profits or healthcare company stock prices.

The revolution continues, but the great news is that its ultimate success will lead to monumental changes in the treatment of diseases we currently fear—the many chronic illnesses that are killing us today will become rare, preventable, and manageable, from neurodegenerative disease to psychiatric illness to inflammatory and autoimmune disease.

This twenty-first-century approach will combine root cause identification for each patient, computer-based analysis of whole genomes and biochemistry, app-based longitudinal functional analysis, and personalized precision protocols to render the currently untreatable chronic illnesses optional rather than inevitable.

The communication guru Marshall McLuhan famously said, "The medium is the message," referring to the observation that we receive information not just from the content of a message but also from the medium itself, whether it be newspaper or television or computer or something else. In the ongoing medical revolution, the medium is beyond print, beyond television, beyond the internet. The medium is healthspan, brainspan, lifespan—indeed, the medium is life itself.

ACKNOWLEDGMENTS

My thanks and admiration go to the thousands of people with cognitive decline who have had the strength and discipline to commit to a comprehensive precision-medicine protocol—you are indeed paving the way for success in millions. Thanks also go to your families, practitioners, and health coaches, who together are easing the burden of dementia for so many.

Thanks also to a superb physician—my wife, Aida, who is always focused on improving patients' lives—and to our beloved daughters, Tara and Tess. Special thanks to Diana Merriam and the Evanthea Foundation for their vision, commitment, continued enthusiasm, and guidance. I am grateful to Phyllis and Jim Easton for their commitment to making a difference for people with Alzheimer's disease. I am also grateful to Katherine Gehl, Marcy, Jessica Lewin, Wright Robinson, Dr. Patrick Soon-Shiong, Douglas Rosenberg, Beryl Buck, Dagmar and David Dolby, Stephen D. Bechtel Jr., Lucinda Watson, Tom Marshall and the Joseph Drown Foundation, Bill Justice, Dave and Sheila Mitchell, Josh Berman, Marcus Blackmore, Hideo Yamada, and Jeffrey Lipton.

Our research on neurodegenerative disease, and its ultimate translation, would not have been possible without the training I received from leading scientists and physicians: professors Stanley Prusiner, Mark Wrighton (chancellor), Roger Sperry, Robert Collins, Robert Fishman, Roger Simon, Vishwanath Lingappa, William

Schwartz, Kenneth McCarty Jr., J. Richard Baringer, Neil Raskin, Robert Layzer, Seymour Benzer, Erkki Ruoslahti, Lee Hood, and Mike Merzenich.

Special thanks to director Hideyuki Tokigawa and director of photography Ivan Kovac of the documentary *What Is Your Most Important Memory?*

I am also grateful to the functional medicine pioneers and experts who are revolutionizing medicine and healthcare: Drs. Jeffrey Bland, David Perlmutter, Mark Hyman, Dean Ornish, Ritchie Shoemaker, Neil Nathan, Joseph Pizzorno, Sara Gottfried, David Jones, Patrick Hanaway, Terry Wahls, Stephen Gundry, Ari Vojdani, Prudence Hall, Tom O'Bryan, Chris Kresser, Mary Kay Ross, Edwin Amos, Ann Hathaway, Kathleen Toups, Deborah Gordon, Jeralyn Brossfield, Kristine Burke, Jill Carnahan, Susan Sklar, Mary Ackerley, Sunjya Schweig, Sharon Hausman-Cohen, Nate Bergman, Kim Clawson Rosenstein, Wes Youngberg, Craig Tanio, Dave Jenkins, Miki Okuno, Elroy Vojdani, Chris Shade, health coaches Amylee Amos, Aarti Batavia, and Tess Bredesen, and the over seventeen hundred physicians from ten countries and around the United States who have participated in, and contributed to, the course focused on the protocol described in this book. In addition, I am grateful to Lance Kelly, Sho Okada, Bill Lipa, Scott Grant, Ryan Morishige, Ekta Agrawal, Christine Coward, Carolina Curlionis, Jane Connelly, Lucy Kim, Melissa Manning, Casey Currie, Chase Kennedy, Gahren Markarian, and the team at Apollo Health, for their outstanding work on the ReCODE algorithm, coding, and reports; to Darrin Peterson and the team at LifeSeasons; to Taka Kondo and the team at Yamada Bee.

For three decades of experiments that led us to the first reversals of cognitive decline, I am grateful to Shahrooz Rabizadeh, Patrick

Mehlen, Varghese John, Rammohan Rao, Patricia Spilman, Jesus Campagna, Rowena Abulencia, Kayvan Niazi, Litao Zhong, Alexei Kurakin, Darci Kane, Karen Poksay, Clare Peters-Libeu, Veena Theendakara, Veronica Galvan, Molly Susag, Alex Matalis, and all of the other present and past members of the Bredesen Laboratory, as well as to my colleagues at the Buck Institute for Research on Aging, UCSF, the Sanford Burnham Prebys Medical Discovery Institute, and UCLA.

For their friendship and many discussions over the years, I thank Shahrooz Rabizadeh, Patrick Mehlen, Michael Ellerby, David Greenberg, John Reed, Guy Salvesen, Tuck Finch, Nuria Assa-Munt, Kim and Rob Rosenstein, Eric Tore and Carol Adolfson, Akane Yamaguchi, Judy and Paul Bernstein, Beverly and Roldan Boorman, Sandy and Harlan Kleiman, Philip Bredesen and Andrea Conte, Deborah Freeman, Peter Logan, Sandi and Bill Nicholson, Stephen and Mary Kay Ross, Mary McEachron, and Douglas Green.

Finally, I am grateful for the outstanding team with which I have worked on this book: for the writing and editing of Corey Powell; literary agents John Maas and Celeste Fine of ParkFine; and editor Caroline Sutton, publisher Megan Newman, and Avery Books at Penguin Random House.

NOTES

Introduction: Lost in Translation

xiv **multiple groups contradict this claim:** Tiia Ngandu et al. (2015). "A 2 year multidomain intervention of diet, exercise, cognitive training, and vascular risk monitoring versus control to prevent cognitive decline in at-risk elderly people (FINGER): a randomised controlled trial." *The Lancet* 385 (9984): 2255–63. doi:10.1016/S0140-6736(15)60461-5; Richard S. Isaacson et al. (2018). "The clinical practice of risk reduction for Alzheimer's disease: a precision medicine approach." *Alzheimer's & Dementia: The Journal of the Alzheimer's Association* 14 (12): 1663–73. doi:10.1016/j.jalz.2018.08.004.

xviii **the FDA released a "smoke signal" statement:** Berkeley Lovelace Jr. "Biogen's stock jumps 42% after FDA staff says it has enough data to support approving Alzheimer's drug." *CNBC,* November 4, 2020. https://www.cnbc.com/2020/11/04/biogens-stock-jumps-30percent-after-fda-staff-says-it-has-enough-data-to-support-approving-alzheimers-drug-.html.

xxi **the "yes if" people and the "no because" people:** Harrison Price. *Walt's Revolution! By the Numbers.* Orlando: Ripley Entertainment, 2004.

Chapter 2. Deborah's Story: My Father's Daughter

35 **I switched to a Mediterranean-style diet:** Note that the KetoFLEX 12/3 diet we developed has advantages over the MIND diet in that it induces ketosis, which is critical for best outcomes in those with dementia, it removes inflammation-associated dairy, and it removes grains that may be associated with leaky gut. Fortunately, Deborah has done very well without adopting all of the components of the KetoFLEX 12/3 diet.

Chapter 7. Julie's Story: Good Luck with That

129 **a paper describing a hundred patients who followed the same protocol:** Dale E. Bredesen et al. (2018). "Reversal of cognitive decline: 100 patients." *Journal*

of Alzheimer's Disease & Parkinsonism 8 (5): 450. doi:10.4172/2161-0460 .1000450.

Chapter 8. Questions and Pushback: Resistance Training

139 **clinical results were published:** Dale E. Bredesen (2014). "Reversal of cognitive decline: a novel therapeutic program." *Aging* 6 (9): 707–17. doi:10.18632 /aging.100690; Dale E. Bredesen (2015). "Metabolic profiling distinguishes three subtypes of Alzheimer's disease." *Aging* 7 (8): 595–600. doi:10.18632 /aging.100801; Dale E. Bredesen et al. (2016). "Reversal of cognitive decline in Alzheimer's disease." *Aging* 8 (6): 1250–58. doi:10.18632/aging.100981; Dale E. Bredesen et al. (2018). "Reversal of cognitive decline: 100 patients." *Journal of Alzheimer's Disease & Parkinsonism* 8 (5): 450. doi:10.4172 /2161-0460.1000450.

Chapter 9. Misconceptions and Misperceptions: Digging In Our Heals

144 **The drugs offer a false sense of security:** Richard E. Kennedy et al. (2018). "Association of concomitant use of cholinesterase inhibitors or memantine with cognitive decline in Alzheimer clinical trials: a meta-analysis." *JAMA Network Open* 1 (7): e184080. doi:10.1001/jamanetworkopen.2018.4080.

145 *Herpes simplex:* Ruth F. Itzhaki (2018). "Corroboration of a major role for herpes simplex virus type 1 in Alzheimer's disease." *Frontiers in Aging Neuroscience* 10: 324. doi:10.3389/fnagi.2018.00324.

145 *HHV-6A:* Ben Readhead et al. (2018). "Multiscale analysis of three independent Alzheimer's cohorts reveals disruption of molecular, genetic, and clinical networks by human herpesvirus." *Neuron* 99 (1): 64–82. doi:10.1016 /j.neuron.2018.05.023.

145 *Porphyromonas gingivalis:* Stephen S. Dominy et al. (2019). "*Porphyromonas gingivalis* in Alzheimer's disease brains: evidence for disease causation and treatment with small-molecule inhibitors." *Science Advances* 5 (1): eaau3333. doi:10.1126/sciadv.aau3333.

145 **a related spirochete:** Judith Miklossy (2011). "Alzheimer's disease—a neurospirochetosis. Analysis of the evidence following Koch's and Hill's criteria." *Journal of Neuroinflammation* 8: 90. doi:10.1186/1742-2094-8-90.

145 **a yeast such as** *Candida:* Diana Pisa et al. (2015). "Different brain regions are infected with fungi in Alzheimer's disease." *Scientific Reports* 5: 15015. doi:10.1038/srep15015.

145 **various molds:** Diana Pisa et al. (2017). "Polymicrobial infections in brain tissue from Alzheimer's disease patients." *Scientific Reports* 7 (1): 5559. doi:10 .1038/s41598-017-05903-y.

147 **"Most experts don't recommend genetic testing for late-onset Alzheimer's":** Mayo Clinic Staff. "Alzheimer's genes: Are you at risk?" Mayo Clinic, April 19, 2019. https://www.mayoclinic.org/diseases-conditions/alzheimers-disease /in-depth/alzheimers-genes/art-20046552.

147 **the FINGER study from Finland:** Tiia Ngandu et al. (2015). "A 2 year multi-domain intervention of diet, exercise, cognitive training, and vascular risk monitoring versus control to prevent cognitive decline in at-risk elderly people (FINGER): a randomised controlled trial." *The Lancet* 385 (9984): 2255–63. doi:10.1016/S0140-6736(15)60461-5.

149 **well-documented examples of the reversal:** Dale E. Bredesen (2014). "Reversal of cognitive decline: a novel therapeutic program." *Aging* 6 (9): 707–17. doi:10.18632/aging.100690; Dale E. Bredesen et al. (2016). "Reversal of cognitive decline in Alzheimer's disease." *Aging* 8 (6): 1250–58. doi:10.18632 /aging.100981; Dale E. Bredesen et al. (2018) "Reversal of cognitive decline: 100 patients." *Journal of Alzheimer's Disease & Parkinsonism* 8 (5): 450. doi:10.4172/2161-0460.1000450.

Chapter 10. Quantified Self and the Reversal of Cognitive Decline

156 **ketones provide an alternative energy source to the usual glucose:** Stephen C. Cunnane et al. (2016). "Can ketones help rescue brain fuel supply in later life? Implications for cognitive health during aging and the treatment of Alzheimer's disease." *Frontiers in Molecular Neuroscience* 9 (53). doi: 10.3389/fnmol .2016.00053.

157 **all laboratory targets are listed:** Dale E. Bredesen. *The End of Alzheimer's Program: The First Protocol to Enhance Cognition and Reverse Decline at Any Age.* New York: Avery, 2020.

158 **direct correlation with brain shrinkage:** Nicola Andrea Marchi et al. (2020). "Mean oxygen saturation during sleep is related to specific brain atrophy pattern." *Annals of Neurology* 87 (6): 921–30. doi:10.1002/ana.25728.

158 **important addition to the treatment of cognitive decline:** Gordon K. Wilcock et al. (2018). "Potential of low dose leuco-methylthioninium bis(hydromethane sulphonate) (LMTM) monotherapy for treatment of mild Alzheimer's disease: Cohort analysis as modified primary outcome in a Phase III clinical trial." *Journal of Alzheimer's Disease* 61 (1): 435–57. doi:10.3233/JAD-170560.

159 **people with Alzheimer's disease are insulin resistant in their brains:** Roger J. Mullins et al. (2017). "Exosomal biomarkers of brain insulin resistance associated with regional atrophy in Alzheimer's disease." *Human Brain Mapping* 38 (4): 1933–40. doi:10.1002/hbm.23494.

161 **which affects 80 million Americans:** Allison Nimlos. "Insulin resistance: what you need to know." *Insulin Nation*, July 25, 2013. https://insulinnation.com/treatment/medicine-drugs/know-insulin-resistance/.

161 **a website called Cronometer:** "Cronometer," accessed January 4, 2021. https://cronometer.com/.

162 **check your hormone levels easily:** Apollo Health. "Cognoscopy," accessed January 4, 2021. https://www.apollohealthco.com/cognoscopy/.

162 **a serum test for BDNF:** Margaret N. Groves. "Exploring the connection between BDNF and Alzheimer's disease." *ZRT Laboratory Blog*, September 20, 2019. https://www.zrtlab.com/blog/categories/bdnf.

162 **cognition-supporting fat, called plasmalogens:** Carissa Perez Olson (2019). "Clinical matters: High-plasmalogen diets and Alzheimer's." *Today's Geriatric Medicine* 12 (5): 6. https://www.todaysgeriatricmedicine.com/archive/SO19p6.shtml.

162 **supplements to increase these levels:** Prodome. "Welcome to Prodome," accessed January 4, 2021. https://prodrome.com/.

162 **Cerebrolysin:** X. Antón Alvarez et al. (2003). "Positive effects of Cerebrolysin on electroencephalogram slowing, cognition and clinical outcome in patients with postacute traumatic brain injury: an exploratory study." *International Clinical Psychopharmacology* 18 (5): 271–78. doi:10.1097/00004850-200309000-00003.

162 **Davunetide:** Michael Gold et al. (2012). "Critical appraisal of the role of davunetide in the treatment of progressive supranuclear palsy." *Neuropsychiatric Disease and Treatment* (8): 85–93. doi:10.2147/NDT.S12518.

162 **thymosin beta-4:** Wikipedia. "Thymosin beta-4." Last modified January 1, 2021. https://en.wikipedia.org/wiki/Thymosin_beta-4.

165 **shown to be an antimicrobial peptide:** Stephanie J. Soscia et al. (2010). "The Alzheimer's disease-associated amyloid β-protein is an antimicrobial peptide." *PLOS ONE* 5 (3): e9505. doi:10.1371/journal.pone.0009505.

171 **Dr. Ritchie Shoemaker:** Ritchie C. Shoemaker. *Surviving Mold: Life in the Era of Dangerous Buildings.* New York: Otter Bay Books, 2010.

171 **Dr. Neil Nathan:** Neil Nathan. *Toxic: Heal Your Body from Mold Toxicity, Lyme Disease, Multiple Chemical Sensitivities, and Chronic Environmental Illness.* Las Vegas: Victory Belt Publishing, 2018.

171 **Dr. Joseph Pizzorno has written a superb manual:** Joseph Pizzorno. *The Toxin Solution: How Hidden Poisons in the Air, Water, Food, and Products We Use Are Destroying Our Health—and What We Can Do to Fix It.* New York: HarperOne, 2017.

174 **stem cells may help with regeneration:** Xin-Yu Liu, Lin-Po Yang, and Lan Zhao (2020). "Stem cell therapy for Alzheimer's disease." *World Journal of Stem Cells* 12 (8): 787–802. doi:10.4252/wjsc.v12.i8.787.

Chapter 11. Adaptation, Application: Might Other Diseases Respond?

180 **poor oxygenation due to sleep apnea:** Tiarnan D. L. Keenan, Raph Goldacre, and Michael J. Goldacre (2017). "Associations between obstructive sleep apnoea, primary open angle glaucoma and age-related macular degeneration: record linkage study." *British Journal of Ophthalmology* 101 (2): 155–59. doi:10.1136/bjophthalmol-2015-308278.

180 **anything that reduces the supplies needed . . . also increases risk:** Vassilios P. Kozobolis et al. (1999). "Correlation between age-related macular degeneration and pseudoexfoliation syndrome in the population of Crete (Greece)." *Archives of Ophthalmology* 117 (5): 664–69. doi:10.1001/archopht.117.5.664.

183 **reduces the detox process itself:** Stephanie Seneff et al. (2016). "Does glyphosate acting as a glycine analogue contribute to ALS?" *Journal of Bioinformatics, Proteomics and Imaging Analysis* 2 (2): 140–60. doi:10.15436/2381 -0793.16.1173.

184 **over 70 percent of patients with ALS:** Hiroyuki Nodera et al. (2014). "Frequent hepatic steatosis in amyotrophic lateral sclerosis: implication for systemic involvement." *Neurology and Clinical Neuroscience* 3 (2): 58–62. doi:10.1111 /ncn3.143.

Chapter 12. Gums, Germs, and Steal: A Pandemic Twofer

188 **a pandemic within a pandemic:** Jeffrey Bland. "COVID-19: A pandemic within a pandemic." *Medium*, June 26, 2020. https://medium.com/@jeffrey blandphd/covid-19-a-pandemic-within-a-pandemic-fd0f4fca373b.

188 **Fascinating research on the origin of the COVID-19 virus:** Jonathan Latham and Allison Wilson. "A proposed origin for SARS-CoV-2 and the COVID-19 pandemic." *Independent Science News*, July 15, 2020. https://www.indepen dentsciencenews.org/commentaries/a-proposed-origin-for-sars-cov-2-and -the-covid-19-pandemic/.

189 dementia was described . . . by Ayurvedic physicians: Dale E. Bredesen and Rammohan V. Rao (2017). "Ayurvedic profiling of Alzheimer's disease." *Alternative Therapies in Health and Medicine* 23 (3): 46–50. PMID: 2823 6613.

189 third leading cause of death in the United States: Bryan D. James et al. (2014). "Contribution of Alzheimer disease to mortality in the United States." *Neurology* 82 (12): 1045–50. doi:10.1212/WNL.0000000000000240.

190 insults such as viral or bacterial infections: Stephanie J. Soscia et al. (2010). "The Alzheimer's disease-associated amyloid β-protein is an antimicrobial peptide." *PLOS ONE* 5 (3): e9505. doi:10.1371/journal.pone.0009505.

191 "long haulers syndrome": Anthony Komaroff. "The tragedy of the post-COVID 'Long Haulers.'" *Harvard Health Blog*, October 15, 2020. https://www.health.harvard.edu/blog/the-tragedy-of-the-post-covid-long-haulers-2020101521173.

191 relatively young patients developing Parkinson's disease: Patrik Brundin, Avindra Nath, and J. David Beckham (2020). "Is COVID-19 a perfect storm for Parkinson's disease?" *Trends in Neurosciences* 43 (12): 931–33. doi:10.1016/j.tins.2020.10.009.

191 cases of Parkinson's that occurred after epidemic viral illness a century ago: Leslie A. Hoffman and Joel A. Vilensky (2017). "Encephalitis lethargica: 100 years after the epidemic." *Brain* 140 (8): 2246–51. doi:10.1093/brain/awx177.

192 remdesivir has shown little efficacy: Ralph Ellis. "Remdesivir does not reduce COVID-19 mortality, study says." *Medscape Neurology*, October 16, 2020. https://www.medscape.com/viewarticle/939289?src=soc_tw_201017_mscpedt_news_mdscp_remdesivir&faf=1.

Chapter 13. Enhancing "Normal" Cognition: Be All You Can Be

194 20 percent of us are on five or more: Mayo Clinic. "Nearly 7 in 10 Americans take prescription drugs, Mayo Clinic, Olmsted Medical Center find." *Mayo Clinic News Network*, June 19, 2013. https://newsnetwork.mayoclinic.org/discussion/nearly-7-in-10-americans-take-prescription-drugs-mayo-clinic-olmsted-medical-center-find/.

198 60 bits per second by one measure: Fermín Moscoso del Prado Martín. "The thermodynamics of human reaction times." Submitted paper, Cornell University, 2009. https://arxiv.org/abs/0908.3170.

198 cognoscopy: Apollo Health. "Cognoscopy," accessed January 4, 2021. https://www.apollohealthco.com/cognoscopy/.

203 chronic stress . . . associated with brain atrophy: J. Douglas Bremner (2006). "Stress and brain atrophy." *CNS & Neurological Disorders—Drug Targets* 5 (5): 503–12. doi:10.2174/187152706778559309.

205 The Keto FLEX 12/3 lifestyle: Pamela Peak. "What is the Keto Flex 12/3 Diet?" *Peak Health,* June 18, 2018. https://icfmed.com/what-is-the-keto-flex-12-3-diet/.

208 The interest in "young plasma": Melissa Pandika (2019). "Looking to young blood to treat the diseases of aging." *ACS Central Science* 5 (9): 1481–84. doi:10.1021/acscentsci.9b00902.

208 removal of "aging factors" by plasmapheresis: Melod Mehdipour et al. (2020). "Rejuvenation of three germ layers tissues by exchanging old blood plasma with saline-albumin." *Aging* 12 (10): 8790–819. doi:10.18632/aging.103418.

209 evaluation of the microbiomes of organs: Marnie Potgieter et al. (2015). "The dormant blood microbiome in chronic, inflammatory diseases." *FEMS Microbiology Reviews* 39 (4): 567–91. doi:10.1093/femsre/fuv013.

210 retinal amyloid imaging: Yosef Koronyo et al. (2017). "Retinal amyloid pathology and proof-of-concept imaging trial in Alzheimer's disease." *JCI Insight* 2 (16): e93621. doi:10.1172/jci.insight.93621.

Chapter 14. The Revolution Will Not Be Televised (or Reimbursed)

211 The American Revolutionary War resulted in the deaths of 37,000 people: Wikipedia. "List of Wars by Death Toll." Last modified January 4, 2021. https://en.wikipedia.org/wiki/List_of_wars_by_death_toll.

INDEX

Also by

DALE E. BREDESEN, MD

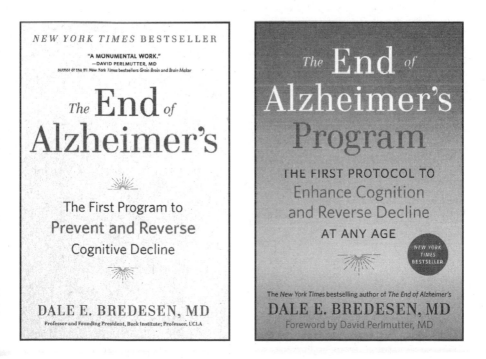